Bertha and Tillie FOREVER

FRAN LEWIS

PUBLISHED BY FIDELI PUBLISHING INC.

Growing up, my sister and I had fun doing many things together. But, like all sisters, we had our moments. I have included some funny stories that really did happen to the real Bertha and Tillie. These are dedicated to my sister Marcia Wallach, my best friend and co-conspirator in everything we ever did and got away with.

I miss you more than words can say.

— Frani

Table of Contents

Welcome to the Wonderful World of Bertha and Tillie

Hi to my young readers, from Fran Lewis, the author of *Bertha and Tillie*. Welcome to their wonderful world! Before writing these short stories, I was a New York City teacher for over thirty years. I taught grades one through six as well as becoming the Reading and Writing Staff Developer for my school. Teaching children to read is really very rewarding and introducing them to writing and creating their own stories was exciting for the students and me as well.

Growing up can be really difficult when you are overweight or not really good at sports or dancing. I hope that you will learn by reading my stories that you can be anything that you want to be and no one can stop you from reaching your goals and dreams. Not everyone is born athletic, beautiful, thin and a genius. But, every one of

you is smart or excellent at something whether it is draw-
ing, jump rope or even running track, it does not matter.
Who you are makes you special. I hope that you enjoy
reading about Bertha and Tillie and learn that there is a
little bit of Bertha in everyone.

Love, Bertha

Bertha and Tillie
FOREVER

We grew up as Marcia and Fran. My sister was thin, had brown hair that she complained frizzed all the time, and could sing and dance better than most stars on Broadway. These are true stories. My sister was like a ray of sunshine on a cloudy day. She always brought out the best in everyone and she never frowned. She had a sunny personality and a wonderful mind. No matter what the situation was she managed to figure out what do. Sometimes the solutions were great and at other times comical. Here are some funny stories that Marcia/Tillie and Bertha/Fran would love to share with you.

Bertha One More Time: I'll Tell It My Way

This book is dedicated to the memory of my sister, Marcia/Tillie who passed away last July. We had some really fun times and wild experiences growing up that I thought I would share them with everyone. She was funny, headstrong, wild in her own way and adventurous. I, on the other hand, was quiet, reserved but dictatorial in nature when necessary. These are all true stories that I hope will make you laugh, cry, cheer for Tillie and Bertha and want to read more. I am going to write these my way and do not worry about the tenses, the word placements or anything else. I want to tell this and relate them to the reader exactly the way they happened.

Tillie: It's Your Turn

"Tillie, Bertha, get in here. Your room looks like a battle zone and I, for one, do not want to pick up the mess. Bertha, you should know better than to throw your books all over the place; and Tillie, what is this with clothes all over the floor and bed and doorknob?"

Tillie: "I am trying to decide what to wear tomorrow. I really need to look my best. I have nothing really great to wear and Bertha is definitely not my size—as you can tell—and your clothes are outdated and old-fashioned. I really need a fashion coordinator or a shopping spree before tomorrow morning. Since there is no way that is going to happen, I guess I will have to use what I have and hope for the best."

Bertha: "Thanks for the great words, Tillie. Even if we were the same size I would never let you borrow anything because you would ruin it, smell it up and never give it back!"

Mom: "Before I do something like ground you both for life, get into that room and put everything away or else you won't have to worry about what to wear. Get my drift, Tillie? Bertha, you too now! Put those books on the shelf, the shoes where they belong and your fashion show back on the rack. GOT IT?"

Tillie and Bertha: Yes, Mom!

Bertha and Tillie's room was really small, and they shared one small closet, but each had their own dresser and shoe rack. Bertha made her bed and Tillie remade hers as Bertha perched herself on top of her blanket and began to direct Tillie as to where to put everything that needed to be put away.

Bertha: "Look Tillie, this room is really too small for both of us to move around in and put things away. Here is what we will do: Working together, I will direct you as to where to put each thing since I never forget where things go and you do. All you have to do is put the items back where I tell you, nice and neat, and then you can go off to your friend Gina's house for dinner, get out of my face, and I can sit on the phone and talk to my friends after I get done with my homework."

Bertha: "That dress goes over there in the back of the closet. The jacket goes in the hall closet, the shoes go under the rack in the hall closet, and the pants get hung up in here. See how easy that is? Next, my books go on the shelf in alphabetical order, and make sure the titles are facing out. Next, the pencils and pens need to go in the desk drawer, and you should fill the printer with paper and a new cartridge so I can complete my homework and not have to search for supplies after I type my report and yours too. Finally, you need to get a broom and sweep under your bed and mine to make sure that there are no papers there or anything else. I will straighten my pillows and yours and then we will be done. Boy, that was easy but really tiring. We did a great job as usual. Wait until Mom sees what we did."

Tillie: "Yeah, right: You direct and I do everything. What teamwork?"

Bertha: "Without my direction and perfect planning, you would never have gotten this done so fast—I mean we would never have gotten this done so fast—and you would not be able to go to your crazy friends for dinner. Bye, Tillie, see you later; or better yet, are you staying over at her house?"

Tillie: "None of your business, big Bertha."

Bertha: "Ma, she called me fat: she is so mean to me. She is always making fun of me because she is so thin and cute, and I am oversized and overstuffed. Well, more for me if you do not come home until tomorrow."

Sisters
But So Very Different

Bertha and Tillie were sisters. Bertha, that's me, and Tillie, grew up in the Bronx and lived in a small apartment over a candy store. On the first floor above lived our cousins Philippi and Theresa. Around the corner in apartment eight lived our other cousin Annie. I was short, pudgy and had a round face that was shaped like an apple. My long black hair was held up in a ponytail. Tillie, my sister, was taller than me and had long blonde hair that always frizzed up when the weather got hot. Tillie had brown eyes and had the look of mischief in her eyes letting you know that she was always one step ahead of you.

I had always been overweight, and I always had trouble losing weight. No matter how hard I tried, the weight never came off. I could eat a celery stalk or just look at something delicious and gain a pound. I guess my body loved food so much it just grew at the sight of it.

I also hated going to school because everyone made fun of me because I was fat. They called me Big Bertha, the big waddling duck. They'd say, "There is Big Bertha waddling down the street," or "Here comes the Big TUBBY." I'd tried to not care and hide my tears, but I couldn't; my face turned a deep red and my cheeks puffed out. My nose, that was already too big for my face, started to twitch and I really just wanted to run away and hide.

My mom chose my clothes and always had me wearing polka dots or stripes, which made me look like a round beach ball. Imagine wearing a red and pink polka dot dress to school with black saddle shoes and white socks. No one wanted to be caught wearing such an awful outfit. But, my mom thought I was cute.

It was in this outfit that I went to school on my first day of sixth grade. Can you imagine what all of the other kids thought about how I looked? Not only did I look like a beached whale in polka dots, but I looked like the poster child for what not to wear in any year.

My cousins, sister and friends were all in the same school and lined up in the morning lineup yard with the fourth graders. My sister, Tillie, was wearing a lovely pink dress with beautiful bows. My cousins were dressed in blue and white jumpers and looked really cute. I hated them and my mom for making me look ridiculous. Just because I was the only plus sized sixth grader didn't mean that she had to make me look even more plus.

As the teachers arrived to pick up their classes and the other children in my class got on line, I saw many of them just staring at me. Some of them started to laugh and some just plain fell on the floor. One of the boys, who was really mean, told the other boys that I looked like his fat Aunt Margie. Another said that I reminded him of his grandmother in that dress. He said she had the same one and wore it to church on Sundays. If that wasn't enough, when we finally got into the classroom and seats were assigned, I could not fit in the small wooden seats and behind the desk. The teacher had to give me a special desk and a bigger chair. Not only was I overweight, but at ten years old I was close to four feet five inches tall. I was so embarrassed I just sat with my head down the entire day and could not wait for dismissal time.

When lunchtime came I went to lunch with my cousins and my sister, only to be humiliated even more by my cousins. They started whispering about me and how much I ate. Even though all I had was a tuna sandwich and an apple, they still thought it was funny and laughed at me anyway. No one was nice or even tried to make me feel better.

When lunch was over, all of the children in the school had some time to play in the yard. I just stood on the side and watched everyone running around, playing punch ball or jumping rope. No one included me in anything, and after a while I felt almost invisible. It was the worst day of my life.

When school was finally over, I told my mom that I never wanted to go back again. I told her what the other kids did and that the teacher made me sit alone in a separate seat because I was so fat. What I did not tell her was that teacher was not very nice to me, and even said that I could use a real big diet to look like the other kids.

After school, since it was the first day, we were allowed to go and get a treat at the candy store. My sister, the skinny Minnie, decided to get a malted with whipped cream and a slice of pizza. My cousins decided to get pizza and some ice cream. I decided to get pizza, ice cream and a malted in order to drown my sorrows in food. I know that it was not a smart thing to do, but then, being only eleven and with no one to tell me how to deal with mean children and people, I did what most people do — I ate until I couldn't eat anymore.

The first week of school only got worse, to be followed by my real nightmare, which was dancing school on Saturday mornings. My mom took all of us to dancing school. We went in her little car, where I was made to squeeze in the back seat with my cousins. Our lessons were in a small hall on Hunts Point in the Bronx. Everyone was excited about these lessons and the upcoming recital; everyone, that is, except me. I hated dancing school. I couldn't stand ballet or acrobatics. I really did not like putting on my leotard when I felt like 160 pounds of jiggling fat and blubber. I could barely fit into the tights, and the leotard made me look like something between the fat lady in the circus and Miss Piggy in a pink ballet outfit. My mom felt that dancing lessons would be good for me and would make me more graceful, and possibly help me lose weight. All it did was make me more self-conscious and want to crawl under a rock or into a turtle shell and hide. But, being so fat, I could not fit into a turtle shell or even a seashell.

After dancing school we were allowed to go out for a treat. I only wanted to eat my way into oblivion and forget my first week in school and the tortuous time I had at dancing school. While everyone was doing ballet or toe, I was busy trying to figure out one simple step in tap. I could barely walk in those shoes without slipping, and I was totally jealous of all the other skinny and graceful people doing toe and ballet.

We went out to our favorite restaurant on Mohegan Avenue for lunch. We loved to go to Sally's for a great sandwich, and then next door to the candy store for ice cream. I ate until I felt I would burst, but of course I had room for ice cream. I figured after all of that dancing and stress I deserved something.

The following weeks in school only got worse. I must have gained at least five pounds eating and trying to make myself feel better. The kids in my class just laughed at me when we went to gym or recess. The teacher wanted us to run around the outer yard and then try to learn folk dancing with the dancing teacher. More torture and more stress! What did I do to deserve this? Oh yeah! I was born fat and was getting even fatter. I was doing this to myself and I did not even realize it. Even running around the yard was hard. I could barely catch my breath after ten seconds, let alone ten minutes.

Even though I was only eleven years old I realized that I could not go on like this anymore. I went to the doctor, who took a lot of tests and finally told me that I had a thyroid problem that was causing my weight gain. He gave me some medication to take, and I began losing some of the weight. But, even with the pills I was never really able to lose that much, and I was never really very agile or limber like my sister and my cousins. So, I gave up trying. I decided to channel my energies into things that I did well, and maybe even better than everyone else in my family.

The first thing I had to do was convince my mom to let me dress the way I wanted. She had to stop picking out my clothes and let me wear what would make me feel prettier and happier. This took a lot of convincing on my part, but with some help from my grandmother I finally won the argument and was allowed to shop for myself.

With this first hurdle accomplished, I next went to find shoes that did not make my feet look so flat and so wide. I was wearing saddle shoes, and they were not very flattering. I found a pair of black shoes that were more like sneakers and had an arch for my feet; and at least they were more fashionable.

I had lost about ten pounds from the thyroid medication and from just watching my diet. I was still overweight but I had a better outlook on things.

The next week, I went to school in my new outfit and even some of the more popular girls said I looked nice. Of course there were those who had other things to say, but I finally decided to ignore them. I know at eleven you are still very impressionable and can get hurt easily, but I decided to toughen up and not care what other people thought of how I looked. If that wasn't good enough for everyone that was too bad.

As I grew up, I realized that throughout junior high and high school things would only get worse. Girls can be really cruel, and boys enjoy making fun of fat girls. I never really got down to the size I wanted to be in junior high or high school. I always had the weight problem, but I wore clothes that I picked out and tried my best to be fashionable.

My sister Tillie went to the same school as me and she was always popular with the boys and the girls. She starred in all of the school plays, and in some she had the lead role. I would sit in the audience and feel proud that my sister had such great talent. I, on the other hand, could play the piano and the violin and would accompany her on the piano when she wanted to rehearse.

Playing an instrument was my way of showing the world that I had a special talent too. I was very smart and always got good grades, but that never really mattered when everyone else did too. In order to stand out and be recognized just for being me, I decided to practice a lot and become first violinist in junior and senior high. I worked really hard and succeeded. It did not matter to my teachers what I looked like, although nerd comes to mind. All they cared about was how well I played in the orchestra and how we would sound in concert. This was the first time in my life that I felt special, and I did not have to be thin or pretty to succeed. Being first violinist also gave me the privilege of using the best violin in the school and sometimes conducting the orchestra.

Being overweight is very traumatic when you are a young child, but it is just as awful when you get older. Throughout my entire young adult life I, Bertha, have fought with a weight problem. There were times when I just ate myself into oblivion and did not care about anything. I became so frustrated that I eventually became so overweight that I could barely walk.

Being short and wearing clothes that were oversized, I hid my weight fairly well, but I knew it was there. My cousins would laugh at me when they watched me eat. They said, "You look more like Tubby the Tuba than Tubby."

They even laughed at me when I told them that I was going to lose weight and really try hard to become thin. Of course, in my heart I knew that this was going to be hard, but try I did. Eventually, I did lose some of the weight when my thyroid was finally under control. However, it did not mean that I could resume my binge eating.

Weight is something that is hard to control, but it can be done. Not everyone is beautiful on the outside, but everyone is on the inside. It is that inner beauty that you need to show; the rest does not matter.

I am no longer overweight. I went on a diet plan that I finally created by myself. It took a long time to see any results. I went from 175 to 110, and I feel great. I still can't dance, ice skate or run fast, but I do look and feel better.

Kids can really be unfeeling when they think you are different or should look a certain way. It is up to parents and educators to make sure that what happened to me does not happen to their students or children. Everyone is special and different. If we all looked alike, the world would be a dull place. It is our differences that make us special and who we really are.

Fran Lewis

The Cooking Lesson that Failed

My sister was a great cook and tried her best to teach me how to impress a date by making chicken Parmesan. However, as hard as she tried and as easy as she made the recipe, there were several ingredients that I'd never heard of — or should I say, misinterpreted — since I wasn't a cook, which makes for my unique chicken parm dish.

Let's start with the simple ingredients:

Chicken cutlets	Salt and pepper
Breadcrumbs	Grated cheese
Olive oil	Mozzarella cheese
Frying pan	One oven
Eggs	Timer
Tomato sauce	Baking pan
Garlic	

She explained how to crack the eggs and said to be careful not to leave any of the shell in the bowl: not as easy as you think. Next was the hard step: olive oil in the pan. I never went shopping for olive oil, so I bought a jar of olives and poured the oil from the jar into the pan, and then rubbed the olives all over the chicken. There, I did it!

Not quite: I needed more liquid in the pan, but I was still not ready to attempt the rest. I never bought bread-crumbs either, so I took Wonder white bread, broke up five slices into little pieces, and put it in the eggs. When I put each cutlet into this mixture, low and behold the pieces of white bread sort of stuck to the chicken, the eggs looked kind of weird, and I was so proud of myself. I put the cutlets into the frying pan, and I could not understand why the white balls of bread and crust came off of the cutlets and the chicken sort of smelled like salty olives.

Next, when I thought they were done, I poured sauce over them, and then a slice of mozzarella cheese and more sauce. I then turned on the oven and set it, as my sister stated in her instructions, for 350 degrees. Oh, before I forget, she did draw a diagram of how to turn on the stove and which knobs would Tilld help me set the oven at the right heat. She even told me to go to the butcher or meat market for the cutlets … like I didn't know that.

The end result was too comical. I took them out and served them with pasta that I made, which turned out not too bad. But, my poor date could not understand what the white marshmallow looking balls were and why they looked like cotton balls; and where were the bread-crumbs? I never did fully explain it.

My Thyroid Hates Me; That's Why I Am Fat!

At ten years old, I was five feet tall and five feet wide. I looked like I had the back end of a truck instead of a cute little booty. I weighed over 160 pounds, reluctantly went to dancing school and exercise class, and I even toppled over when trying to ice skate and crushed the poor instructor. If that wasn't bad enough, tourists in New York visiting the ice skating rink in Rockefeller Center photographed *me*. I was not a really big eater, except when I was aggravated, agitated or pressured to get straight 100s on all of my tests; I never really pigged out, except when necessary. But, my sister, skinny little Tillie, could eat anything and everything and never gain weight. She was taller than me, prettier and could really dance and sing. I, dear poor Bertha, was awarded the klutz awkward and overweight award at the ripe old age of ten. So, what does this have to do with my dear old rotten thyroid? EVERYTHING!

I was determined to lose weight in spite of myself. I really did not overeat, and I just did all of the wrong things all of the time. But, even when I watched what I ate and did not eat any candy, sweets or junk foods — except for Cracker Jacks, which were too hard to resist — I still did not lose weight. So, I needed to narrow it down and figure out who was to blame … something else or me!

My favorite person in the whole world was my grandma Katie. She was so smart and understood me better than anyone else. I waited until my mom and my sister went to Alexander's to go shopping for clothes. I loved shopping, but not when I was forced to try things on. My sister wore a size four and I was a sixteen. My mom, Rose, liked us to wear the same dresses in different sizes. Now, think about that for a minute and do not crack up too much. You see, my sister picked out the dresses that she liked which had stripes and polkadots, and I had to wear the same thing. How, horrific is that? Just picture it in your mind! Better yet, DON'T!

When the coast was clear I went into the kitchen where my grandmother was making her famous chicken soup from scratch. I told her my problem and asked what she thought I should do. For one week, she made dishes that were clearly not fattening and were healthy for me to eat, hoping that I would lose at least one pound in one week. Instead, I gained three more. I did not cheat and

I ate only what she prepared, even at lunchtime. We did this for two more weeks, then Grandma suggested that I see our doctor. She trusted that I would not cheat, and I did not.

Not telling anyone where we were going, we headed for Dr. Ballot's office and made him promise not to tell anyone why we were there; better yet that we had even come there. He was probably the best diagnostician and doctor in the whole world. Doctors today do not care so much for their patients, make house calls on demand, or really speak to both the kids they treat and the adults, explaining what they find and what can be done to cure or fix the problem. He did all of the tests necessary and listened to what we had tried. He said he knew what the problem was, but I would have to come back and take a basal metabolism test to check my thyroid function. Well, I now had something to blame besides me … I hoped!

Taking the test took quite some time, and I had to lie still with all of these tubes in my nose and more. After the test was done he stated that my thyroid was sluggish and underactive at least 17%, and that would account for the weight gain and other things that affected my hormones. He explained that I had to take medication to speed up my thyroid and regulate it. But, unfortunately, he had to spring this on my mom first She understood and was not mad or angry that I trusted my grandmother on this project and not her. My mom never had a weight problem either, just my dad … but he liked to eat.

As a result of taking the medication, I did lose some weight. However, the medication made me nervous, jumpy and irritable and it had to be adjusted. Thyroid problems have plagued me all of my life. It can become a serious issue if not taken care of. I could not understand why I was so tired, sluggish and achy all of the time, or why I was gaining weight. These are just some of the symptoms of having hypothyroid disorder. Not fun.

Years later, I was diagnosed with Grave's Disease, which is just the opposite of hypothyroid disease — it is hy*per*thyroid disease. Your thyroid is overactive and running in speed zone. Not fun either. I was really agitated, angry, mean, and confrontational, could not stand up straight, could not even walk up steps without my legs burning. The end result was another trip to the doctor and more pills. These helped me to slow down my thyroid, but increased my weight by at least fifty pounds; even though I was watching my diet, the doctor said it would not help. Needless to say, when my thyroid was regulated and I finally stopped taking the pills I was thrilled.

So, you see, my thyroid really hates me, and that explains why I was overweight and fat all of my life. But, I'm not fat anymore. I took off all of the weight I gained from the pills and then some. I get my blood checked every three months, and although I have made friends with that little gland in my neck, I hope we remain on neutral terms forever and I never have to take pills again.

Be nice to your thyroid: You do not want it to turn on you. Get yourself checked out and stay healthy.

— Bertha

Family Day:
Finally Bertha's Choice

First there were dancing lessons, and next ice-skating lessons. These were followed by violin and piano lessons. What was going to be next? The next torture my mom and my sister Tillie had in store for me was roller skating lessons! Is there no justice in the world? Why was it that everything I did had to be related to weight loss and exercise? Why couldn't we do something on the weekend that required using your intelligence and thinking skills? Why couldn't we do something that everyone in the family wanted to do, and not just my sister Tillie?

I really did not have the answer to any of these questions, but I could try to change their minds by reminding everyone of what happened when I went ice-skating in Rockefeller Center. I tried really hard to skate and kept falling on top of my instructor, who solved the problem by giving my dad his money back for the entire lesson. Did they really think that I would do better at roller-skating? I didn't think so.

We started out for the roller rink on Kingsbridge Avenue in the Bronx when I had a brilliant idea. Why didn't we get tickets to watch the New York Chiefs and the Boston Bombers in the roller derby instead of going roller-skating? My sister thought this was an awful idea because she thought roller derby was boring and too violent. I loved it. I was not a great skater, I did not want to take roller skating lessons and have the same embarrassing incident I did when I went ice-skating. One disaster should be enough for anyone. But, Tillie, the sports oriented and more coordinated of the two of us, got an A on her Spanish test and she won. Poor me, I got an A on all of my tests that week, yet once again I was forced to go along with the majority. But, I was not going down quietly this time.

When we arrived at the roller rink I saw my cousin Annie and her father Harry there. Annie did not like to roller skate and my uncle loved roller derby almost as much as I did. I asked my parents if I could go watch the skaters in the roller derby instead of skating myself, but they said they did not want Tillie to take lessons all alone. They felt that we should always do family things on family day together. How unfair was that! Family day was supposed to be for everyone, not just one person.

I went over to the desk to get my skates and they gave me a pair of size fives to fit my flat feet. I put them on and attached the skate part with the skate key, and tried to stand on them by myself before meeting my instructor. This time I was determined not to be embarrassed and not to fall on my rear end in front of everyone in the rink. I was finally able to balance myself by holding on to the beginners bar on the side of the rink. I tried to walk in the skates and did not fall. I tried to glide and fell right on my face and heard a loud rip. Not again, oh please not again!

I was wearing my brand new black bell-bottom pants and a great black and white shirt that I just bought with my own money at Helds on Tremont Avenue. I could not believe that this happened again. I felt a draft coming from behind me and knew that I had split my pants. They were not too tight on me, but when I fell I must have fallen on something sharp on the ground near the side of the rink, and whatever it was ripped my pants. I was so disgusted. Why couldn't they just let me go to the roller derby where I would enjoy myself?

Well, low and behold, just like in bowling, my mom, Rosie, thought that she would come to the rescue with another one of her fix-its. She had a large sweater with her in case she got cold and she said it was long enough to cover the rip in my pants. I told her that I did not want to take the lesson with a rip in my pants and that I was afraid they would rip more. There was a sports store in the skating rink, so she bought me a pair of sweat pants that I could change into for my lesson. Now, I looked like a big black panda bear with my black pants, my black and white shirt and the awful sweater that had white fur on it. I looked stupid.

My instructor was a young guy who took one look at me and was about to laugh at my outfit when I shot him a look. I took off the sweater and felt that I did not look that bad, but not great. His name was John and he told me that he could teach anyone to roller skate and he wanted to get started. My dad had paid for an hour's lesson and he wanted to make sure that he got his money's worth. HA HA! FAT CHANCE!

John tried showing me how to stand properly on the skates and how to move my feet from side to side. That did not work. The only thing I could do was ask to hold on to both of his hands and try and not fall on top of this poor man like I did when I took my ice skating lessons. But, this guy was really mean and said that he would never want anyone my size to fall on top of him. and tried helping me over to the railing to hold on. But, as luck would have it, as I tried my best to get there I fell on my side, split my pants that were already too tight and crawled to the seats behind the rink. I took off the skates, threw them at the man at the desk and walked out into the hallway never to return again.

I guess that's not exactly the grown up thing to do but I was totally embarrassed. Kids were laughing at me, including everyone I came with except my sister, Tillie, would not let anyone hurt my feelings. When she saw what happened she came out trying to make me feel better and said the next time she would help me. There was never going to be a next time. But, something good did happen. We were in the rink in the armory and I love roller derby, but I never expected some of my favorite team players on the New York Chiefs to come and practice there. When Gerry Murray and some others came over to me I had no idea that they saw what happened and the way the instructor treated me. Along with them came the manager of the rink, and he made the instructor not only apologize to me for hurting my feelings and not helping me skate, but he said that he would give me ten free lessons too, which I gave to my sister. I took the free tickets to the next five roller derby matches. So, family day turned out to not so bad after all.

Adults can be mean and so can kids. Not everyone is sports-oriented, but some of us try harder than others. Some of us realize our limitations and work from there. I am Bertha. I am smart in school. I play the first violin in the orchestra and I play the piano. My sister can dance, sing, entertain and stars in Broadway shows. She is really amazing. This is Bertha: whatever your talent might be, go for it! You never know!

Bertha and Tillie

Bertha's Fitness Plan

My name is Bertha and I am now twelve years old and still quite overweight. My mom has decided to send me to a weight loss camp, run by my Uncle Jason, for the summer. I am at least thirty pounds overweight for my age and height, and I really need a strong regime of exercise and diet in order to try and get in shape for next year. I am entering middle school and I really want to look good for the boys that might be in my class, and not get laughed out for being fat. Being picked on for being obese and not being able to walk down the street without having trouble catching my breath is starting to get to me.

The only problem with this plan was that I would have to go to Florida in order to be part of my uncle's camp and weight loss program. What a hardship that would be to spend two whole months away from my sister Tillie and my nagging mother and father! I thought that I just might survive and even lose some weight. After convincing my parents that this might be the best way for me to kick-start a weight loss program, they decided to let me go.

My mom called my uncle and his wife, Tammy, to tell them that I would be coming to Florida to go Uncle Jason's weight loss camp. She called my aunt to check on my flight arrival and to find out who would be picking me up at the airport. When that was settled they discussed the camp, the program and their goals for me. I was really annoyed that my mom had to interfere with everything that I did. Since my uncle was a professional trainer and owned his own gym called Body Solutions in Plantation, Florida, I think that she should leave it up to him to worry about the program.

After they finished their phone call I began packing for my two months away. I decided that I needed some new clothes, and they agreed that some proper workout clothes would help, along with the proper walking and running shoes that I would need when I ran the track or worked on the treadmill. What I did not know was where this camp was, and what else I was in for. I thought that I would be staying with my aunt and uncle and my cousins Cade, Carly and Casey in their house, but I found out differently.

I left the next morning and arrived in Florida to be picked up by my uncle with some other kids, and we were packed in a bus that said 'Body Solutions Weight Loss

Camp for Overweight Children. How embarrassing was that? Right there in front of everyone in the whole airport was this huge bus with this huge sign telling everyone that we were overweight and needed help. The other kids did not seem to mind because they were ready to start their program and the road to being lean and mean. I, on the other hand, stuffed my hand inside the pocket of my jacket and ate a Milky Way bar as fast as I could just to fortify myself with what was going to come. I did not want to start the program feeling weak and undernourished.

We arrived at the camp and were taken to wooden huts and given our bunks and weight buddies. We were told that we had one half hour to unpack before lunch, and then we'd be starting our training. At that point I knew that I needed another sugar boost, because exercising could really make you weak and tired, and without sugar I might not be able to keep up. Good thing I had another Milky Way Bar and two Almond Joys.

We all entered the lunchroom hut and were seated next to our weight loss buddy. My buddy's name was Sally Jo, and she must have weighed at least 300 pounds and really needed this program. Next to her were Marcy and her buddy Lara Lee, who must have been the thinnest person there and looked like she did not need the program at all. She said that her mother had enrolled her in a modeling agency and she needed to lose twenty pounds or she would not get any shoots or jobs. In order to work for the agency you had to be really thin.

My Uncle Jason came in and introduced himself, and started to tell us about the program and our daily schedules. I got tired of just listening and started to daydream and drift off, when he came right up to me and told me this was not the way to a great start. He told me that if I did not get with the program I would be sent home and someone else would take my place. He gave us the rest of the afternoon to get to know the other children and get settled. If lunch was an indication of what was to come, I was glad I was prepared with my own food and my own idea of a weight loss program.

After lunch we were each assigned a weight loss coach who would outline our daily programs and our fitness schedules for the week. My luck as usual…I got the oldest person on the team, who looked about fifty years older than everyone else and reminded me of an army drill sergeant. As he outlined my program he told me things would only get tougher and I would really have to work hard every day in order to get fit. He told me I was one of the most overweight kids in the whole program and I really needed to lose weight. Added to that he said I had nothing else to offer anyone because I looked like I could not do sports or any other physical activity. I felt like quitting before I started. Instead, I smiled politely at

Mr. Ugly and decided that I would create my own brand of torture for him. But, first I felt myself fading away and needed some reinforcement. I asked to go to the bathroom and downed three Hershey Bars before coming out and starting my torture.

The first thing he wanted to teach me was how to do deep knee bends. Did you ever see a hippo dance, or try to bend down and pick something up? Did you ever see a giraffe try to bend over? Just imagine a 170 pound kid shaped like a hippo who was about 5 feet 4 inches tall trying to bend and not able to. As I tried to bend just my legs, my behind stuck out behind me and I fell over on my face. I tried again and again and could not bend straight down, so he had to hold my waist. stick his knee in my back and practically gave me a wedgy before getting me to do one deep knee bend the right way. I felt so exhilarated after doing one whole deep knee bend. I bet that I lost at least five pounds just doing that. I was so proud of myself, I tried to do one more so that I would have done an even two deep knee bends. What a great feat for the first time.

After doing a second deep knee bend I thought that I would be rewarded with a break. No such luck. He wanted me to do at least twenty more before going on to the next exercise, which was leg stretches and ab crunches. Just the thought of twenty more deep knee bends and ab crunches made my blood sugar decrease and let me know that it was snack time, not crunch time. Well, maybe Crunch Bar time.

I started to do the knee bends, and on the tenth one my left knee locked in place and I could not get up. He had to straighten out my leg, and boy did that hurt. He told me to try again until I was had done the twenty, letting me know that just because my uncle owned the camp did not mean I was going to get special treatment. As a matter of fact, since my uncle was his boss, he was going to make sure that I lost more weight than anyone else in the program. It was at this point I knew that I was going to have to come up with a plan of my own to escape some of this torture and pain.

After completing the knee bends and attempting to do the leg stretches, I knew that ab crunches were out of the question. I was so sore and so tired that the only thing I needed was a Crunch Bar and some Coke to restore my energy level. Thank goodness they did not know where I had hidden my stash.

I asked to be excused to go to the bathroom before starting on the crunches. I took the long way and headed for the locker room, where I knew I would be able to go to the bathroom and find what I needed in order to exist. I looked around to make sure I wasn't followed, and found the bag that I had hidden away in the locker room with my personal survival kit. I ate three Crunch Bars and one Tootsie Roll and felt so much better. I rinsed out my mouth with some water to make sure that there would be on remnants of any chocolate for him to see or smell.

I left the locker room and returned to my instructor, who told me that I would have to do double for taking so long. If I had known that I would have eaten double to increase my energy level.

He showed me how to do the crunches and I could barely do one. I tried to do an entire crunch and he realized that I could barely sit up. He showed me how to do half crunches, which were also too hard for me to do. He put his hand on my back and pushed me up, and showed me how to lower my neck. I did one and then asked if I could try again the next day. He made me do five before allowing me to stop. But, I was not done yet. I had to do fifteen minutes on the treadmill before I was allowed to quit for the day. That at least I could do. How hard could it be to let the machine do the walking for me? I forgot that I had to walk on the treadmill and be able to keep up with the speed that he chose for me.

When that was over he told me to get cleaned up and get ready for dinner. If lunch was indication of what dinner would be, I would certainly waste away real fast.

I went to the dinner hut and sat down next to some girls that I did not know. We introduced ourselves and proceeded to discuss the programs that we had followed that day. Some of the girls were really excited about what they were able to do. I pretended to be happy, but all I felt was sore and very frustrated. I guessed I would have to do better the next day. My uncle was the owner of the weight camp. How would it look if his niece gained weight?

The next day and the day that followed were the same. I tried to do the knee bends, I walked on the treadmill and I even did five ab crunches. But, when it came to jumping over the horse or the parallel bars, I was a complete failure. Holding on to the bars and walking across them without someone holding on to me was impossible. I could not lift myself up off the ground, so he had to have three people help me reach the bars and keep my legs off the ground. I could not jump over the horse — I would run up to the horse and freeze in front of it. Even jumping high enough to sit on it was too much for me. I thought the instructor was going to have to come up with some other ways to help me lose weight.

I tried really hard, but nothing seemed to be working. I even cut down on the amount of candy I snuck during the day. I was going to get serious about this and really try to lose weight. But, at the end of the first week, with cutting down on the candy and eating the seaweed, salads and low calorie food each meal, I only lost one half of a pound. I guessed that was better than gaining half a pound. But, my instructor was disappointed and told my uncle that I might need a different kind of exercise program to lose weight. He suggested that instead of knee bends I would walk around the track for thirty minutes in the morning and thirty minutes in the afternoon. I thought that might work. He suggested that jumping rope might be better than the knee bends and the treadmill. He also suggested that maybe since I liked to swim that would be better than the ab crunches. That sounded like something I might be able to do.

We decided to start my program the next morning. I got up and had a small breakfast of oatmeal, cereal and one chocolate bar. I really needed to start off on my diet tapering slowly. I didn't want my system to go into "lack of sugar shock."

The instructor started by showing me how to use a jump rope without strangling myself. I tried to jump without getting tangled in the rope and was not able to do it at first … I was not jumping high enough to clear the rope. I tried and I tried but I still could not jump high enough and my legs kept getting tangled in the rope. He decided to try something else. He had me just jump up and down in place as if I was on a trampoline. I began jumping higher and higher and I felt that I might be getting somewhere. He decided to try the rope again and this time I was able to do three jumps before getting tangled up again.

I did this all afternoon and the best I could do was ten jumps in a row. I guess that was good because my drill instructor did not look too unhappy with me.

Next, we moved on to swimming. He wanted me to do at least three or four laps the long way. The pool was an Olympic size pool but I was not and will never be an Olympic size swimmer. I am not a good swimmer, so doing that many laps and getting out of breath real fast was not going to work. I needed to take baby steps or baby laps. He decided that swimming the long way was not the answer. I could not make it from the deep end to the shallow end without having to stop. My legs were heavy and they started to cramp as I got to the center of the pool. He decided that it would be okay if I swam the short way. I was able to do the three laps because the distance was shorter and I felt some kind of success at last.

After completing my swimming session I was allowed to take a ten-minute break before having to work on the treadmill. My instructor told me that I would begin with a twenty- minute workout on the treadmill and work up to forty-five minutes before the end of the week. At this point, even though I felt successful at swimming, I knew that I would need something to help keep up my strength, and I knew that eating chocolate and candy was not the answer. I asked him if he had any fruit or something that would boost my energy level so that I could keep up with the day's program. He handed me an energy bar and said that would help. It really was quite small and didn't taste great, but it was better than candy.

I went to work on the treadmill and he set it at a medium speed to begin my workout program. I was able to handle the entire twenty minutes by listening to the music in the gym and pretending to know how to dance to the music, or in this case walk. At the end of the day, I felt that I had really accomplished something, and knew that by the end of the summer I would be thinner and in much better shape.

I worked hard the entire first week and could not wait to get on the scale to see how I had done. Everyone was gathered together in the gym where they had several scales. Each instructor had ten students that they were working with. What we did not know was that we were in competition. The group that lost the most each week would be given a day off to go into town to see a movie, have a healthy meal at a restaurant, and a day of shopping for a new outfit for the end of summer award dinner. Everyone was excited about this, but I guess it would have been nice to know that we were in an actual competition and not just an exercise program. I think I definitely would have been more motivated not to keep sneaking my treats if I'd known what was at stake. Unfortunately, the group that gained weight as a group or lost the least was in for a rough time.

There were five groups of ten students. Each group got weighed individually and then each group got weighed on a huge scale as a group. How embarrassing was that. The first group of ten weighed 1,500 pounds as a group. The next came close to 1,600 pounds, and the third and fourth were tied at 2,000 pounds. My group came in at 2,100 pounds and lost. The average weight of each person in our group was 210 pounds for some of the boys; I came in at 155, and had lost five pounds and felt great. The rest of my group gained weight. As a result we could not have any snacks at dinner, nor could we have a free day. As a matter of fact, they decided that instead of individual instruction, we would now work out as a group. I was really upset about losing and went straight back to my hut and ate three candy bars. I was fuming. Here I tried my best and lost weight, only to be a loser again.

The next couple of weeks I did not even attempt to do my best. I worked out with the group and followed what my instructor had to say, but when the day was over and I had eaten all of their meals, I ate my own treats to make myself feel better and so did my teammates. We were a team and got along really well as long as someone provided the midnight snacks for the rest of the group.

At the end of the first month, our group had lost ten pounds as a group, but still had the lowest amount of weight lost. I even gained back my five pounds, which made my Uncle Jason really upset, and he let me know it. How did it look if the niece of the director of the camp gained weight and did not make him proud by following the program? He even said that I should set the example for the rest of the students and lose the most weight. Now, I thought he was pushing it, but I would definitely try harder. That meant that I would have to stop sneaking the extra treats and stop having those late night snacks with the other kids in my group. But, even more, I would now have to convince everyone in my group to do the same thing without telling them that I was the niece of the director.

That night after we had our steamed chicken with steamed vegetables and a small salad for dinner, we all headed to our hut for the nightly talk with our instructor about the events of that day and what we planned for the next day. He had decided to work with us as a group and not individually, putting more pressure on everyone to follow the program and be a real team.

The next morning, we got up and had breakfast. The first activity was going to be a two-mile hike in the woods followed by a forty-minute workout on the treadmill. After that we would have a light lunch to be followed by a short swimming lesson. We would then have to do ten laps across the pool and then have a short talk about our progress for that part of the day. The rest of the day I could practice my jump rope skills, learn to use the StairMaster and take a step-class. By the end of the day, I could barely move, and I knew that dinner was not going to be enough for me. I also knew that I needed more than a candy bar to keep up my strength, but I held out and went for extra fruit at dinner.

The following day was the same as the day before, except that new things were added. Now, we had a three-mile hike every morning, a twenty-lap swim and a two-hour workout in the gym. I was getting better at exercising, but I really did not know if I was losing weight. After all, I tried and tried, but I could not resist that extra potato chip, tortilla chip or anything else that might help fortify me. It was a good thing that I packed one suitcase with snacks and clothes. It was even better that no one ever found out.

It was the last week of the program and it was coming down to the wire. On Friday, we would gather in the gym and be weighed as a group and individually. Our weights and weight loss or gains would be read out loud for everyone to hear. This was not going to be good. The last week of the program I tried really hard and ate practically no extra snacks after ten o'clock at night. I hoped that I'd lost some weight. I really did not want to face my family, especially my sister Tillie and my mother, if I did not lose some weight. I would never hear the end of it.

On the final Friday before we all went home, we had a special celebration followed by the big weigh-in. All of the groups lined up together with their instructors in front of five different scales that were brought in just for that day. The first group went on as a group and had lost 150 pounds. Since there were ten in a group, the average weight loss was about fifteen pounds. The next two groups went on and they lost 200 pounds as a group. The last two groups were mine, and one other. The other group lost 300 pounds as a group. The average weight loss was about thirty pounds. That was really impressive.

My group was last. All I prayed for was some weight loss for the group and not a weight gain. Since we had the lowest amount of loss all summer, I knew that we would never win the prize for losing the most weight and get the grand prize of a $500 gift card to go shopping for new clothes. That was the final incentive for each group to try their best. Every member of the group would get this $500 Visa Gift Card. The student that lost the most weight would get one too, even if that person was not in the winning group.

My group got on the scale and everyone started to scream. Some of the other kids started to even laugh. I could not see the scale but I knew once again that we came in last. Our final weight loss was 100 pounds. We came in last, but we did not gain any weight. Our average weight loss was about ten pounds. Then, they weighed everyone individually to see who lost the most weight.

When it came to my turn, I had lost only eight pounds the entire summer. But, I looked better. My legs were firmer from the exercise, and I had lost one size in my dresses and my pants. Things were finally a little big on me. I was thrilled and felt that even though I cheated, I still managed to lose some weight. Of course, my uncle was not thrilled with my results and he could not understand why I had not lost more. But, we won't tell him or anyone else, will we?

The next morning everyone was herded back onto the bus from the camp and driven home, or in my case to the airport. I was really disappointed. I thought I would spend some time with my cousins, Dani Nic, Kati Rose, Carly Megan and Casey Dallas instead I headed directly for home.

When I arrived home my mom took one look at me and cried. She was sure that I would gain weight, and I think she was finally proud of my effort to try and slim down. I really should have tried harder and not eaten the extra snacks that I brought. But, all of my life, everyone had never really had any faith in me to lose weight until my Uncle Jason invited me to his camp and the instructor tried to help me. I guess if I had been in a group that was more motivated I would have lost more. But, I really can't blame anyone but myself.

For anyone who has trouble losing weight and gets invited to join a kid's weight loss program — DO IT and DO YOUR BEST TO SUCCEED. I am going to try and continue to lose more weight. If you have any weight loss problems or stories to share with me, please write me and let me know. I will try and answer your letters.

Love,
Bertha

I Am Beautiful, I Am Me

Not everyone in the world is born beautiful or pretty. I certainly was not. I was born fat, with a big nose, long black hair that never stayed in one place and a huge bottom that could be seen blocks away even before I arrived where I was going. My name is Bertha; I am ten years old and this is my story.

I grew up in the Bronx and lived in an apartment building over some small stores. I have a sister named Tillie, and I call her skinny Minnie behind her back. Tillie, my sister, was taller than me and had long blonde hair that always frizzed up when the weather got hot. Tillie had brown eyes and had the look of trouble in her eyes letting you know that she is always one step ahead of you.

I had gone through a huge growth spurt, and was now one of the tallest children in my class. Those made me stand out even more because not only was I oversized but tall as well. McDonald's has their super sized meals and I have me the only super-sized ten year old in the world.

Lunchtime came around and we were all herded into the lunchroom. My mom would not let me eat school lunches. She packed our lunches or brought them to our classroom before we went to eat. My mom, Rosie, was the PTA president of our school and she could come and go as she pleased. If she wanted to watch me in class she could. But, that is another story.

On this day she had made me what she called a good lunch. At this point after suffering through school and being laughed at, all I wanted to do was eat my way into oblivion and not worry about the rest. She made me a tuna sandwich with lettuce. She labeled it in case she thought I didn't know what I was eating. She placed some carrots that were also labeled, in foil, with celery and some tomatoes. I, on the other hand, had already taken a bag of chips and had them hidden in my school bag in case I need comfort food to make me feel better.

When we all sat down to eat at lunch one of the girls in my class, Frieda, asked me if I wanted her sandwich too. Frieda was tall and thin and really pretty. She was laughing as she asked me if I wanted to eat half of her ham and cheese and finish the rest of her snack. She said "You look like that would not be enough for you since you are so fat, and what is worse not pretty at all."

I looked at her, grabbed her sandwich and threw it on the floor, got up, and walked out of the lunchroom. How grown up was that? Instead of standing up for myself I backed away because I was embarrassed.

Everyone is not pretty, like I said at the beginning of this story. Everyone is good at something that will make them stand out. However, up until now the only thing that made me stand out was my big nose, big bottom and my wide body. I decided to get noticed another way. I decided that I would show everyone that I was good at something other than eating. That's when I really started working hard on my music, and I excelled!

Because I was focused on practicing my musical instruments and was doing really well, I decided to give dieting another try. I did not tell anyone what I was doing except the one person I could trust, my grandmother, Katie. She was the only one that I could talk to, and who understood my problem. She was the smartest person in the world to me and she tried to help me deal with the mean kids too.

Grandma took on the job of preparing lunches and creating healthy dinners for me too. I started to have oat-meal or cereal with skim milk in the morning. At times, she would make me egg whites or egg white omelettes to make sure that I had a good and healthy start to the day. She would wait for everyone to leave for work or school before preparing my lunches and breakfast. This was our special secret.

For lunch she made me salads with a can of tuna packed in an ice pack so it would not spoil. She would make boiled chicken and make me a sandwich with mustard and lettuce. She would grind her own chicken to make me a cold chicken burger and added carrots and celery stalks plus a can of seltzer.

For dinner she made me salmon with spinach or grilled chicken or some type of white meat chicken or turkey. She even made me the best chicken soup in the whole world. Grandma even made her own pasta noodles with egg whites and not eggs so I could eat them with some tomato sauce.

Bertha, that's me will never be beautiful and never be gorgeous. But, I will never be overweight again. In six months I lost ten pounds, and in one year I lost over twenty. I ate grapefruit for snacks and other fresh fruit too. I never ate chips any more, and rarely had ice cream or cake. Once in a while, I would have a slice of thin crusted pizza with a salad.

The best part was, for the first time in my life, Bertha, that's me, was thinner and weighed less than my sister, Tillie, and my cousins too.

When I went back to school the following year I started junior high and many of the same children were there. Some of them could not believe how much thinner I had gotten, and others were just as mean as ever.

"Bertha," they said, "You will never ever be really thin, and you will never be pretty. You will always be Bertha the Tub." I did not care what anyone thought. I knew that I had done something none of them could ever do. I just answered them and said, "I might not be pretty on the outside, and you might not want to be my friend, and I don't really care. But, I am me and who I am is more beautiful on the inside than you will ever be." I smiled and walked away. Yes, me, Bertha, stood up for myself and there was no turning back. By the end of my first year of junior high, with the help of my grandmother and my willpower, I weighed 115 pounds and wore a size six.

Bertha, Tillie, Tony and Maria: Friends Forever

Bertha and Tillie loved to go to Luigi's to get their hair done. Luigi's was an upscale salon in the Bronx run by Luigi, John and Gigi. But, Bertha would only let one person do her hair, and that was Tony. Tony was really hot and all the clients wanted him to do their hair. Bertha was older now so she hoped Tony would like her, but he had a crush on Maria.

Maria was really pretty and petite. She worked in the salon as a manicurist and everyone wanted her to do their nails because she was so pretty and hot. She even had male clients with standing appointments, not just because she was so great at her job but she was great to look at too.

Bertha, that's me, had no chance with Tony. True, I had just lost tons of weight, but it did not hide my huge nose that took up half of my face. Tillie, my sister, loved the way Gigi did her hair. Her hair is one huge frizz ball, and he had the magic touch to straighten it and make her look hotter than she already was.

Maria and Tony always looked forward to when we came to the salon. My mother Rosie always brought along treats for everyone even if they were on a diet and did not want the homemade cakes my grandmother made, or the tons of hot chocolate she carried with her in a huge thermos. When Rosie wanted to do something, nothing stopped her.

One Saturday when we were all together, just sitting and talking after our hair was done, Tony and Maria said they needed to talk to us. One of the customers was really hot for Tony and she kept saying horrible things about Maria to Luigi. She wanted her to get fired, and they wanted to know if we could help them get rid of this awful liar. Her name was Dana and she was tall, thin and was a health and fitness instructor. She was constantly offering Tony free passes to her gym, but looked at me and said nothing would work so I should just give up.

Tony smiled at her when he saw her. He even did her hair three times a week. But, no matter what Maria did and how nice she tried to be to her, Dana made up lies about her. One time she said Maria purposely used the wrong shampoo on her hair. Another week she said she got covered in dye when she had her roots done. This week she had said when Maria washed her she'd gotten Dana all wet, and her shirt was ruined. Luigi believed her for some reason—maybe because she was the client, and the customer was always right—but deep down he had to know she was just jealous of Maria and her friendship with Tony. Maria was really worried that she was going to get fired if we did not think of something real fast to teach Dana a lesson.

Revenge is sweet sometimes, and we started to formulate a plan that would work but not in the salon. We decided that one good or bad turn deserves another, and we went to her gym when she was not there and took out six-month memberships. They offered us free training sessions, one free month, and help with any of the machines we wanted to use. The classes in aerobics were great and the instructor seemed nice, until Dana walked in one day and saw me there with Maria. She turned red in the face, stormed over to her boss, and asked what these hoes were doing in her gym. Mind you, she just worked there, and the other instructors were shocked but not surprised at her attitude. But Dana had a way with her boss named Frankie, and she thought she would get away with the same antics she pulled in the hair salon.

Dana sauntered up to Frankie and put her arms around his neck and started to nibble on his ear. But, Mariana, his girlfriend, was there and would not stand by and watch her manhandle Frankie. Mariana walked over and gently removed Dana's hands from Frankie, and then twisted her arm behind her back and threatened to break it if she dared to do that again. Dana, trying to look innocent and coy, looked at Mariana with her steel blue eyes and told her she totally misunderstood, and that she wanted Maria out of her sight because she was after her man, namely Tony.

What happened next was right out of a wrestling match, as Maria decided to not take it anymore and landed the first punch. The next thing we knew they were both wrestling on the floor, and no one seemed to want to stop them. Mariana was coaching Maria and Dana just looked battle scarred by the time all was said and done. Pulling arms, legs, punches, bloody noses and broken ribs, the end result looked worse than a boxing match. When Frankie finally pulled them apart with his assistant Dominick, he pulled Dana into his office, and you won't believe the end result. Angry, fired and definitely not looking her best, she stormed out of the gym aiming to get even with everyone.

Tillie and I called Tony and told him what happened when Maria and I went to the gym to work out. Tillie was fuming when she saw Maria, and she had a fit about what Dana said to me. Tony was not thrilled that Maria needed stitches in her hand, or that Dana got away with just some cuts and bruises. Dana's revenge was just starting, since she got fired and was determined to return the favor to Maria. But, Maria had backup. She had us, and she knew that no matter what Dana pulled we would have her back and take action.

Dana walked into Luigi's as if nothing had happened the previous Saturday. Sidling up to Tony and trying to come on to him, he pretended to enjoy her advances. Tony did her hair and then asked to see her alone in the back room. Whatever he said or did to her no one would ever know. But, the expression on her face said it all as she stormed out of the salon. The smug look on her face was gone, and the ice in her eyes was so cold she could freeze the meat in a locker all by herself.

The next day when Maria was coming to work Dana tried to ambush her before she arrived. Little did she know that someone else was watching her. Dana was fired from her job, but managed to convince the owner of a not so great gym to hire her on as manager. Thinking she now had it made, she wanted her revenge on Maria. Pretending to forgive her, she offered Maria a cup of coffee as a peace offering. But, something told her not to drink it. Thanking her and pretending to believe Dana wanted to remain friends at least because of Tony, Maria took the coffee and did what any forgiving person would do...

dumped it all over Dana and watched it splatter all over her face.

But, Dana would not be looking in the mirror anymore. Dana did not expect Maria to throw the coffee back at her. She'd laced it with acid, and the end result you can only imagine. Maria never meant to hurt anyone but her anger got the better of her, thinking it was just hot coffee. This is a definite twist of events. Maria, Tony, Bertha and Tillie: Friends Forever.

Revenge may be sweet but in this case it backfired. Will Maria get Tony? Well maybe one day.

Family Photos

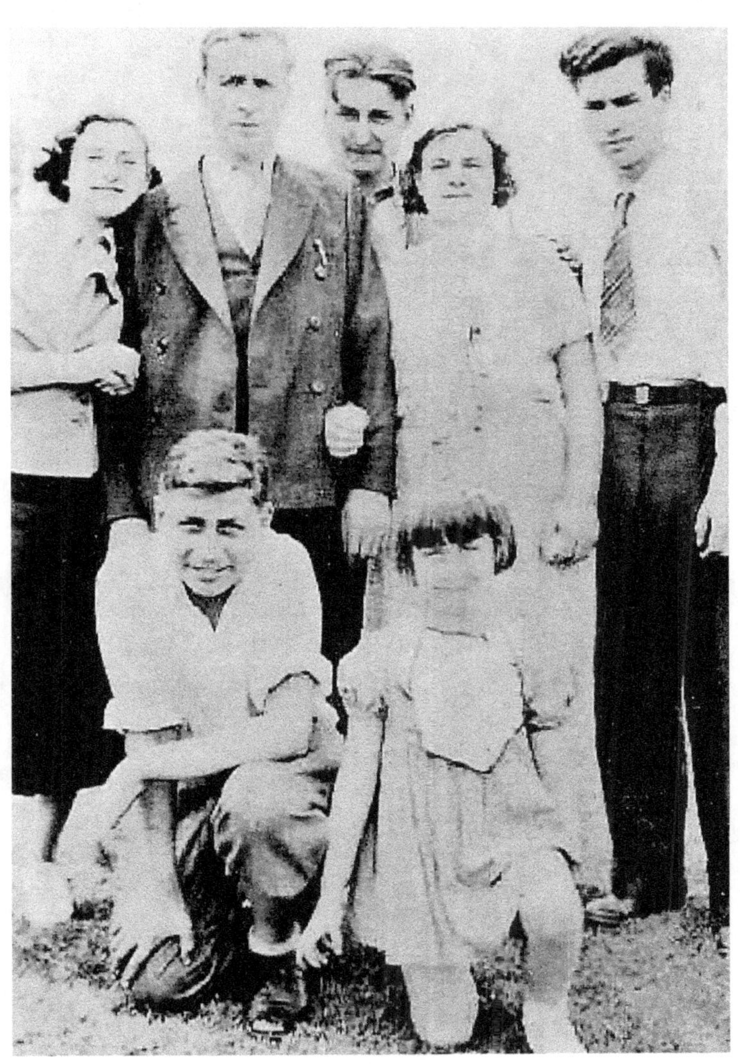

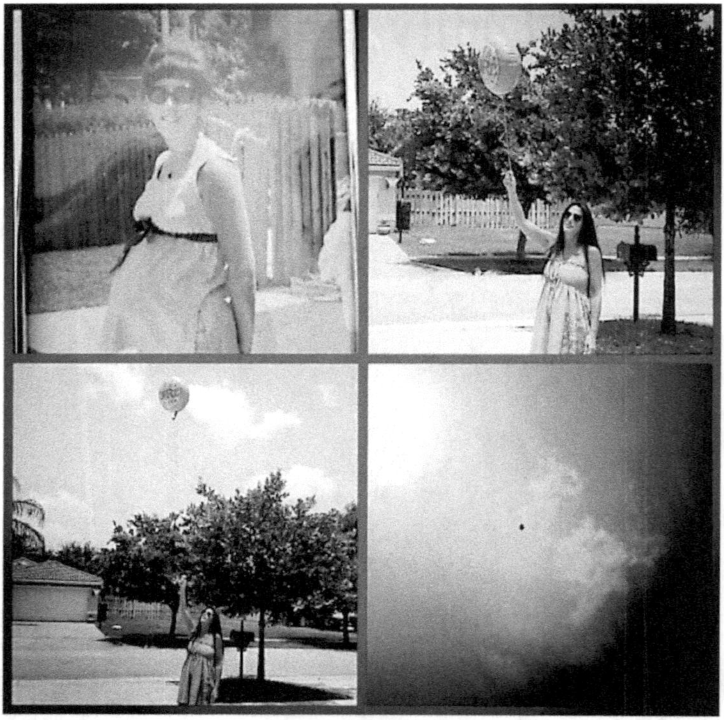

The picture on the top left is my sister, the ones on the top right and bottom left are my niece, her daughter.

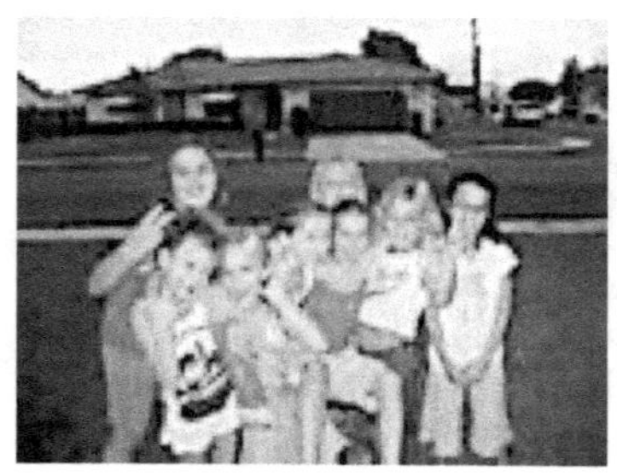

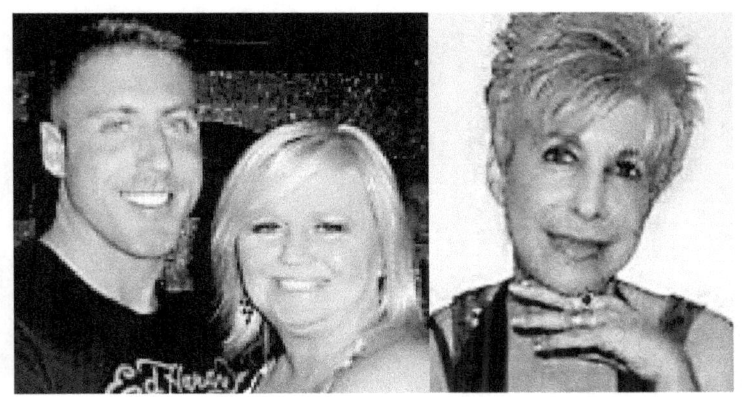

Fran Lewis

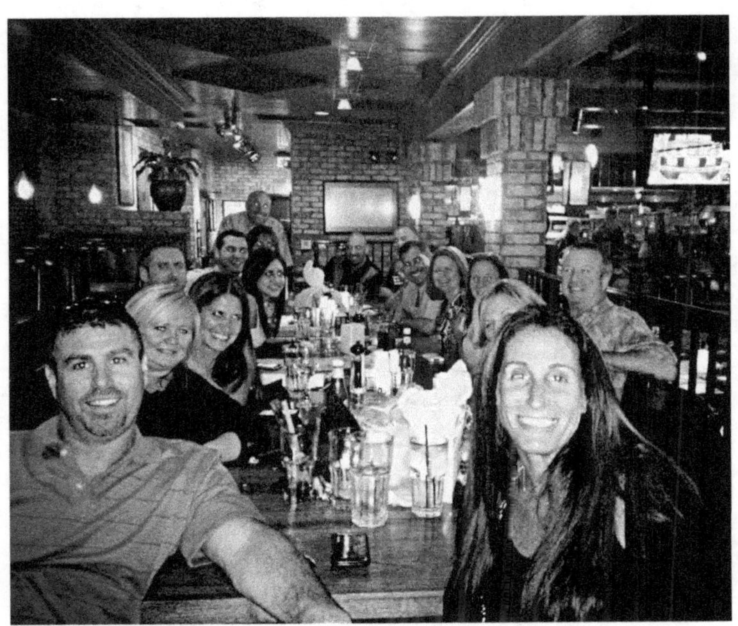

My sister's daughter Jamie and her husband Rob.

Mistakes are Okay, Except If You're Bertha

Dear Readers,

This story is dedicated to all those students out there who try their best in school and still don't succeed in the eyes of their parents. I, Bertha, always study for tests and never hand in an incomplete assignment. I always study for tests, unlike my sister, Tillie, who only has to glance at the information and remembers it. I study for days when I know that I have a test, especially in social studies and science. I have written this to let parents know that when a child does his or her best, even if they don't get 100% on every test but get A's or B's, they should still be proud.

Love,

Bertha

I am Bertha. I have a really hard test today in science and another one in math. I studied for at least four days for each test, and I think I know just about everything in order to get a good grade. Now, you ask why that would be a problem that is causing me to get a big fat migraine headache. Well, it's my mom Rosie; she has decided that I have to get perfect scores on every single test that I take. That means that anything less than 100% is unacceptable.

It started when I came home with my first social studies test in the fourth grade. It was on the first five chapters in the book, which covered about 150 pages of information. My teacher also included the notes that she gave us in class. The test had fifty multiple- choice questions on the Revolutionary War, five essay questions on the causes and results of the Civil War, and the rest were short answer questions based on both wars. My teacher chose these topics for the test and we had to compare the way the colonists handled both wars, and we discussed the different causes and results of both.

Learning the information was really hard but, but I am organized. I sat in my room and had cards with the causes and results of both wars on one side and the people involved and what they did on other cards. The rest of the important information was on the rest of the cards. Oh, yeah, since I am an overweight food freak and I needed my energy, and having a major test, I decided to fortify myself with chips, candy bars and other assorted sweets on my bed in order to help keep up my strength. This was only for the first test; I had not started on the science, which was the same day.

Having four days to study, I broke it up into studying two days for each test. When I had completed my studying for the social studies test, the real torture began. If you think that my dancing and skating lessons were miserable and awful, studying for a test was even worse. After I finished studying my mom, Rosie, would test me on all of the information and have my aunt, who was a teacher and lived next door, come up with questions that I would have to answer as if they were on the real test. This was how my migraine started. If I did not get all of the questions right she would make me look in the book and copy out the answers until I got a perfect score on the test that my aunt had created.

Next, of course, came the science test, and once again I created study cards on the planets and weather, which were the two chapters on this test. I fortified myself with four slices of pizza, five Milky Way bars and went down to the candy store and got a chocolate malted to make sure that I had enough energy to study. Too much sugar is not really good for you, and I would not recommend doing this, but I had to sustain myself for what would come next.

When I was done studying my mom followed the same procedure as she did with the other test and once again I had to complete the test my aunt had created. This time I got all of the questions right and did not have to do anything extra. Did I mention that besides having to study for these tests, I had other homework to do, and violin and piano lessons and practicing as well? My headache only got worse, but I was ten years old and what could I do? The pressure was really mounting up and I knew if I brought home a grade lower than 100% I would really hear about it.

The day of the tests came and I was really scared, so scared that I, Bertha did not even hear what the other kids in my class were saying about me when I walked to class line. I am extremely overweight and I really do care about that, but studying for these tests put such pressure on me that I did what I always do when faced with a problem and stress … I ate. I went to class line, and having grown to being the tallest girl in the class I went to the end of the line. No one really talked to me; they just laughed at my outfits and my ugly saddle shoes and strange hair dos that my mom created daily. I had long black hair that could really have been pretty if she had let me style it in a more modern way. Instead, I had to go to her hairdresser, who did not usually do kid's hair, and suffer with the results.

We went to class and we all sat down while the teacher took attendance. When she was done she handed out the social studies test, and that was when I broke out into a cold sweat, started to shake and almost fainted. I had to really calm down, but being eleven I had no clue what to do or how to take the test, much less get a perfect score. I looked at the first question and my mind went blank; as a matter of fact, I could not remember anything at all. I knew if I came home with a zero or did not take the test I would be in for a lecture and speech from my parents that would take at least ten years to finish. I finally had the solution. I knew that eating in class was not allowed, but what was one piece of chocolate to make a person feel better? So, I broke a rule and took a chocolate kiss from my pocket and ate it. Thank goodness no one saw.

I looked at the questions again and sailed through the test and hoped I passed it. I finished the last essay just about one minute before she called time. No one even realized, not even the teacher, just how nervous I was and what had happened. I don't know if that is good or bad, but at least I took the test without passing out on the floor from fear. Being my size I probably would have put a hole in the floor too and had to pay for the damages.

We took a break for about ten minutes before the teacher gave out the science tests. This test was shorter than the last one, and all I needed to survive were three chocolate kisses that I ate during the break and four candy bars covered in chocolate. I guess the way to calm me down was eating candy and not caring about what the other kids said. But, it did not help my migraine, it only made it worse.

The rest of the day was a total blur for me because my head was pounding so hard I could barely keep my eyes open to concentrate on the rest of the day. I knew that after school I had a violin lesson and then a piano lesson. Then, I would have to tell my mom what the questions were on the test and how I answered them. Hopefully, she would not have time to do a full cross examination, because I had other homework to complete as well. NO SUCH LUCK! My mom was on full battery charge and after my lessons and completing my homework, she made me sit down and tell her what was on the test and how I thought I did. Fortunately, the teacher took her time grading them and I would not know my grades for at least two days.

During this time I had to take an extra dancing lesson to practice for another recital, but this time I was not dancing; I was going to play the piano for the dancers and be spared the embarrassment and misery of having to actually dance in front of 500 people. Next, I had to take two extra piano lessons to make sure that I knew all of the music from memory for the show. That was not hard, it was actually fun.

The next day in school I thought that I would absolutely not survive. Who would have known that my teacher, Ms. Mencher, would decide to mark both tests in one night and not even spare us the pain for another day. She decided to make us suffer until the afternoon to find out our grades. This, of course, caused me to go on an eating binge at lunch since my sister, Tillie, my cousin Annie, and I and were allowed to go out on Friday's for lunch. I ordered two sandwiches, three sodas and of course some dessert to make me feel better, just in case I did not get 100% on both tests. My headache got only worse and I could barely hear what my sister and cousin were saying at lunch. All I did was eat and eat and eat until I felt like I could throw up, and I did just that, all over the floor of the restaurant and all over myself.

Of course, my sister and my cousins were not too happy with what I had just done and were totally embarrassed and pretended not to know me. To make matters worse, I still had to go back to school and face the music, which means getting my test scores on both my social studies and science tests.

I went into the bathroom and did the best I could with cleaning myself up. I was lucky that I had on a sweater and a shirt under it. I took off the dirty sweater and threw it in the garbage. I was not going to carry it with me into the school. I put on my blazer, tucked in my shirt, and rinsed out my mouth, and prayed that no one would notice what I had done or realize what had happened. I also knew that my sister, Tillie would not tell anyone what happened, but I was not so sure about anyone else.

I walked back to school by myself and into the outer yard. The lunchroom teacher, Mr. A, just stared at me and told me I was late and to stand against the wall with all of the late kids. I guess my sister and my cousins never told him what had happened, which was good on one hand, and bad on the other. Now, I would have to face him and the principal for being ten minutes late for school after lunch.

He lined all of us up and marched us into the principal's office. One by one he questioned us to find out why we were late. When it came to my turn, all I could do was cry. I was afraid of him because all he ever did was yelling in your face and scream at you if you broke a rule. But, somehow I got through it and told him what had happened at lunch and why I was late. Of course, my excuse sounded lame, yeah! I was late because I got sick and threw up all over myself, and I left the evidence in the bathroom of the restaurant. But, it must have been the way I said it, and the fact that I was never in trouble and my mom was the PTA President that saved me. He sent me to class with a late pass and an explanation to my teacher. Now, I had to hope she did not read the note out loud for my classmates to hear.

Fortunately, she did not read the note, but did say she was about to return our tests and was going to give them out in order of the highest to the lowest scores. This would be embarrassing for those who received their papers at the end.

Now, I had to pray that I had gotten a perfect score on both tests, and would not have to endure my mom having me write the test over until I knew what I had done wrong and got a perfect score. She said only two children got 100% on the social studies test and three on the science.

I was one of the students who got 100% on the social studies test, but only 98% on the Science. What else was going to go wrong? I could not believe it. Now, I could not go out and get a treat at the end of the day with every-one else; I would have to sit and rewrite my test because I lost two points for what I don't know. I looked over my test and realized that she had given fifty multiple- choice questions each worth two points each. I looked the paper over to see where I had gotten one wrong and lost the two points. She had marked the paper with a 98 but I had made no mistakes. Now, all I had to do was find the courage to tell the teacher that she had added wrong and made a mistake. I had two choices; keep my mouth shut like I always do, or finally speak up so I would not have to rewrite the test for no reason, or have my mom speak for me to get the grade changed.

Well, after this miserable day, and all the studying I had done to get a good grade much less 100%, I raised my hand and told the teacher in a nice way that she had incorrectly scored my test and that I, Bertha, had gotten 100% percent on the test just like the other three students did. She just glared at me and told me she would take off twenty points if I was wrong. I went up to her desk, my face was white, but I stood my ground because I knew that I was right. She looked at me and smiled and said, "Well, Bertha, you finally did it. You did get a 100% on this test, and you spoke up for yourself. I guess you will be doing that from now on. Won't you?" I just nodded my head and smiled after she changed my grade to 100% percent.

Going home I had finally gotten rid of my migraine because I would not have to endure my mom's speech of why-didn't-you-get-a-perfect-score, or have to rewrite the test.

For anyone out there that has this problem, know that after a while I finally told my mom that I would always get good grades, but not everyone gets 100% every time. I thought it was unfair to make me write over an entire test when I had studied real hard and did not deserve to be punished when I got grades over 90%. She was not quite happy with what I had said, but she compromised. I only had to write over the parts that I got wrong. Hopefully, that would not be many things in the future.

No one that studies for a test and tries hard should be punished if they do not get 100%. Children need to be encouraged to do their best and not be afraid to take tests, and certainly should not get headaches like I did.

Love,

Bertha

Are We There Yet?

I hated riding in a car. I really hated riding in the back of a car. Why did I hate riding in a car, you ask. I have always gotten car sick. Not only did I get car sick, but the poor person sitting next to me had to hope that I had good aim when I finally did get sick and spiledl my guts all over the inside and outside of the car. I had told my parents and my sister, Tillie, that I needed to sit in the front seat of the car, or at least next to a window, but no one listened to me. I told them that I should not eat anything before traveling for long periods of time, but no one heard me until it was too late.

It all started every year when we went to the country for summer vacation, and this year was no exception. We piled into my dad's car and headed for April's Sunrise Cottages in Monticello. The first half hour was fine; we played word games, sang songs, and counted how many cows and horses we spotted along the way.

When we had traveled about one hour my Dad decided to stop at the Red Apple Rest for lunch. I told my parents that I was beginning to feel nauseous and should not really eat a lot, but Dad said that it might take until dinnertime to get to our destination, and he knew how much I liked to eat. I did like to eat, but I really didn't want my lunch to be a car decoration for everyone to see when we arrived at our summer home. I really didn't need my cousins to start laughing at me when they saw my lunch all over the outside of my dad's car. But, I was only eleven years old, and I had to listen to my parents. So, I ate lunch and dessert just to teach them and everyone else in the car a really good lesson. "Listen to Bertha when she says that she should eat lightly before traveling, or pay the consequences." After eating a grilled cheese sandwich and fries (my favorite lunch), I ate a salty pretzel and washed it down with a chocolate egg cream. I had bought some Milky Way bars to keep me happy during the rest of the trip. They'd asked for it, and they would surely get it for not listening to me.

After lunch we all piled back into my dad's car, and I asked my sister, Tillie, and my cousin, Annie, to let me sit near a window, and they would not. I sat squashed in the middle between my skinny sister and my not so skinny cousin. Although, she was not as heavy as I was, at 160 pounds she was no lightweight either. This made it doubly hard for me to get any air in the back of the car, even though they opened the tiny window. After riding for about fifteen minutes I told my dad that if he did not stop really soon, the back of his car would be covered with my lunch and so would everyone back there. He told me there was not a shoulder on the road, he could not waste time stopping, and that I should just take some deep breaths and I would be fine. Not really. I could not help what happened next. My sister, Tillie, was sitting next to me on the right and I leaned over her to get to the window to try and poke my head out in order to get some air. But, I missed. I threw up all over her, the outside of the car, the back seat, and myself, of course. I'd warned them, but no one would listen to me. My sister was fuming because I threw up all over her new outfit, and she really wanted to look great when her friend Harvey saw her for the first time this summer. Oh, well. Next time let me sit near a window, and don't be mean.

Poor Annie was covered too. When I put my head back inside, I could not help but try to lean over to her side of the car, and did it again. She was really angry because she wanted to look nice for Harvey's brother, Phillip. Since I had no one to look nice for, I really did not care. Except, I knew that my cousins would be waiting for us when we got there, and I knew that they would be laughing at me because I threw up all over the outside of the car and on my sister and my cousin.

When we finally arrived about an hour later, we had stopped at the nearest gas station and everyone had tried to clean up. Unfortunately, we could not hide what I had done to the outside of the car. My sister was glad and so was my cousin, because they were mad at me for ruining their new outfits and because they had to change into something else. TOUGH!

My cousins were waiting at the top of the hill for us to arrive, and when they saw the outside of the car they fell over laughing, and so did everyone else that was standing there. When we got out of the car they walked over to my sister and my cousin and told them how sorry they were that they had to ride in a car with Barfing Bertha. That really made me angry. I thought next time I would take my own car service, or wait for my grandfather to drive up with my grandmother in their truck.

After all of the laughing stopped and everyone greeted everyone else, I went to my room in my bungalow and refused to come out. My mom Rosie and my father Doc told everyone to just let me cool off. I locked the door to my room and refused to let anyone in until they apologized for making me feel bad. There were a lot of people who got carsick. Why should they make fun of me for getting sick on long trips? On the last trip to the country my cousin, Annie, had gotten really car sick, and we had to take her to a hospital for treatment. But no one made fun of her … just me.

Every Friday or Saturday I helped my father by count-
ing out the money that he'd made all week. I added up his
receipts, and straightened out the money that he carried
in different paper bags. I loved doing this, and I really
liked helping him. It was fun to see how much money he
made every week and how he was doing.

When I finally calmed down and felt better after a
short nap, he came into my room and asked if I would
count the collection, or money, from the store for that
week. I was thrilled to do it. He did remind me that I was
going to be alone in the bungalow because everyone else
was going out, that I should not let anyone inside, and
should keep the door locked. I did just what he said. I
locked the door and bolted it behind everyone.

I went to the table in the kitchen and put all of the
paper bags and the receipts on it. I even lowered the
blinds in the bungalow and double locked the back door.
Even though it was safe, some of the colonies were having trouble with burglaries and I was not going to take a
chance with my dad's money.

When I was sure that everything was secure I opened
the bags and began straightening the money and placing
each domination in different piles. After working on this
for about a half hour someone knocked on the back door.
I ignored it and pretended that no one was there. All of a
sudden I heard someone trying to open the door and ask-

ing if my grandparents were there. I still pretended not to hear them. I hid under the table and did not answer the knock when I heard them yell, "It's us." I had no idea who "us" was and still did not answer. Instead, I took the piles of money and neatly tucked them back in the bags. I began looking for places to hide the money in case someone broke the door and forced it open. I looked in the freezer and there was no room. I thought that might be a good place to hide the money but I was afraid it would freeze. I looked under the bed, which would have been a good idea, but I thought it would be the first place a thief would look. Then, I came up with a real brainstorm. I decided to put the money in the oven. I knew it was off and I put it in the bottom because there was room.

I heard a loud knock, and this time I looked out and saw that it was my aunt and uncle. I opened the door, and told them that I must have been sleeping and never heard them knock. I forgot about the money. They stayed for a few minutes and went back to their bungalow.

I started to read a book, then remembered the collection. Unfortunately, the events to follow were not good. I went over to the oven and opened it up, to be greeted with a huge wave of smoke and the smell of paper burning. I looked down at the bags that had the money and saw them on fire. I took a huge pot, filled it with water and put out the fire, but it was too late. The entire collection went up in flames, and my life was doomed. My parents would probably disown me for being so stupid. I never realized that the bottom of the oven had a pilot light that was always on. I did not think that the money would burn in an oven that was off.

I sat down and did what I always did when I was stressed out. I ate ten candy bars to make me feel better, but I didn't. I started to cry and was really scared. My Uncle Harry was staying in the bungalow next door and must have smelled the smoke, because he came to see what had happened. He was really upset and told me that I should have known better, and I had done a really stupid thing. Well, that made me feel even worse. No sooner did he say that then my parents came in, and I knew that life as I knew it would be over.

They went to the oven, took out the ashes, and placed them on the kitchen table. They said that only half of the money burned, and that by pouring the water I had saved the rest. They also said that some of the burned money could be sent to the U.S. Treasury Department, and they would replace it if they could read the serial number on what was left of the bill, or the amount of the bill. All in all they lost about $6,000 dollars in cash because of my carelessness.

They took the ashes, placed them in a box and put a letter inside of it stating what I had done, and then they had to get it notarized. Now I would be famous in the drug-store where they had it notarized, and the laughing stock of everyone in the bungalow once the news spread…and it did. My cousins made sure that everyone knew what a dumb thing I did, but my sister, Tillie, defended me. She said that it could happen to anyone, and I was just trying to protect the money in case someone tried to break into the bungalow and steal it.

My parents were not happy and told me I would never be allowed to count the money again or work in the store. They felt that I should have known that the oven was always on. I had never cooked in my life, or used a stove. My grandmother and my mother cooked, so how would I know anything about a stove?

While I was out the next morning the other kids called me Firebug Bertha. They kept chanting it all over and over again. I just glared at them. It was a mistake and I felt really bad.

My parents sent the ashes and the small corners of the bills that could be salvaged to the Department of the Treasury in Washington. They waited about two weeks and finally received a letter from them and a check for $2,000. They lost about a total of about $4,000 because of my inexperience. I felt awful, and of course no one understood more than my grandmother. We sat down and talked about what I should have done, and why what

I did was not really stupid, but not so smart either. She made me realize that I had not committed a crime, but an accident along with poor judgment. I felt even worse even though she tried to make feel better by making me my favorite dessert of chocolate pudding with double whipped cream and cherries.

After speaking to her I went outside to try and get into the punch ball game that we played every night. Even though I was the best hitter and could punch a ball farther than anyone else, I was not sure that anyone would let me play, or even want me to play. They said that because of me the entire bungalow could have burned down, and worse. Now, they were being melodramatic. I had put out the fire before it could spread or get any worse. The money was in the bottom of the oven and the only thing that could burn was the bags and the money.

I went over to where the game was being played and saw that my sister, Tillie, was the captain of one team and Philip the other team. My sister told everyone that I was going to play on her team and if they didn't like it, too bad. I felt better knowing that my sister and my cousin Annie would not let anyone make fun of me for my mistake. She told everyone if they didn't like that I was playing that was too bad.

The game was great and my team won. The score was twenty-five to three. I could really punch a ball when

I was angry. It was better than eating myself into fatso oblivion. I was thrilled that we won and that the other team lost, because they were making fun of me for burning the money.

The rest of the summer was great and we really had a fun time until I had to go home. Remember, I got sick on long trips and I knew that this one would not be any different. If they didn't let me sit near a window, they would get what they did on the trip coming up here!

Love,
Bertha

Remember: Accidents happen and people do things that they don't always mean to do. Never put paper in a stove. Never put money in an oven and certainly don't open the door for strangers.

Middle School: Poor Bertha

As if elementary school was not bad enough, now I had to endure the ridicule, misery and torture of going to middle school — more teasing, more picking on and even more name calling by the mean kids who did not like me. In elementary school there were girls who were tough, but not as tough as the group that I met the first day of middle school. They seemed to run things around there, and I mean run them. Even the teachers backed off when they walked through the halls.

Everyone in the school was separated by grade, class, and oh, yeah, clique or group that you belonged to. The girls in my grade, seventh, were not allowed to talk to the ones in the eighth or ninth grades, because we were considered not worthy of being in their presence. We were lowly freshmen, or fresh meat as they called us.

Walking in the school for the first time was really embarrassing; you see, my mom was the PTA president, and she decided to walk her child to school and up to her homeroom the first day. How sad was that! I think that at eleven years old I was quite capable of walking to class by myself. Added to that, she was on a dress code kick and decided to buy me my first day of school outfit. Yes, I, Bertha, who now weighed a little over 150 pounds and was trying to lose weight, was made to wear the ugliest, most unflattering red suit in the whole world. What was even worse, it was made of polyester. Who wore that in this century or any other? The skirt was bright red and was really wide at the bottom, and the waistline was too tight. She bought it a size smaller than I usually wear, just so she would not have to take it in a size if I lost enough weight. This lovely skirt and the awful red and black shirt that went with it made me look like a cross between a wide red apple and a blushing baby hippo. Humiliating and embarrassing, and it got even worse. She even made me wear my ugly saddle shoes, which were also red and really wide and made my feet look like banana boats. All you needed was to put the word *STOP* on my backside and I would be used as a sign to stop traffic.

As I walked into the room I saw many of the kids from my old sixth grade class. They looked human in their outfits. They even had their hair styled with streaks and highlights. I, on the other hand, had begged my mom to let Tony do my hair but she said, "You have lovely black hair, and a ponytail would look cute on you for the first day of school." So, I wore my ponytail and a cute red ribbon over the rubber band. I tried to feather my bangs so that I would somewhat hip — not hippo.

Some of the girls just stared at me and covered their mouths to hide the giggles and snickers. The boys started to make snorting noises and pig sounds when I walked by. After a while, when they saw that I did not show that I cared or didn't get upset, at least outwardly, they stopped.

Next, came our homeroom teacher, Mr. Lee. He was older than most of the other teachers, and you did not want to cross him. He introduced himself, gave out the requirements for his English and social studies programs, and then sent us to the gym. That is where the real misery and horror began.

In this school all of the kids in our class stayed together for every subject. We marched around as a group—or me by myself all day. Walking into the gym, I had on my green gym uniform and my sneakers. I could feel everyone's eyes on me, especially the girls in the other class that we were going to play against. Unfortunately, we had to play with the seventh graders and not a class on our grade level. We were supposed to be the goody two-shoes of the sixth grade, and were hopefully going to spread some goodness into the seventh grade's worst behaved and most evil bunch of girls the school had ever known.

Our gym teacher was young and really afraid of her own shadow, and could use supervision too. This would make what was to come even worse.

When we entered the gym we were separated from the boys in our class and made to line up on one side of the gym facing the girls from the other class. Not only were they older than us but they were known to be the toughest and meanest girls in the school.

The gym teacher, Ms. Strawberry, stood in between both groups of girls and asked for two volunteers, one from each class, to be team captains. No one in my class would raise their hands…they were all afraid to even play. The game was called dodge ball or KILL. The rules were simple. You had to hit the person on the other team to get them out.

Normally, in real dodge ball, you aimed for below the knee and could not hit anyone in the face or chest. In this game there were no holds barred. The girls in the seventh grade were in charge, and the gym teacher was too afraid to stand up to them and let them know who was supposed to be in charge.

So, two girls from that grade were chosen, or volunteered, to be captains. We were told that the teams had to be mixed and were from both classes. The captain of Team One was Dani Nic, a really tough looking blonde with long hair and six earrings in one ear and five in the other. The captain of team two was Casey Dallas, a really tall blonde girl who did modeling on the side and could really play dodge ball. Not only that, but these two girls could just stare at you and make you want to cry.

They proceeded to pick their teams and of course, I was left out. Who would want a 160 pound blimp on their team? I was elected to decide who was out. Now, that was a dangerous job. If I tried to eliminate anyone from the seventh grade I might not make it out of sixth. But, I was not going to let those two scare me, Bertha. At least I thought I wasn't.

The game started and everything seemed to be going okay. Naturally, the only ones I eliminated were from the sixth grade or my class. But, then things got ugly. One girl on Dani's team named Kati Rose accidentally-on-purpose tripped a girl on Casey's team named Carly Megan, and a real fight broke out. Kati Rose and Carly Megan were both in the seventh grade, but no one cared. This was Kill or Dodgeball and they took no prisoners.

Dani walked up to the girl on Casey's team named Genesis, who had pushed Kati Rose and knocked her down. Genesis got up and pushed Mary Rose, who was on Dani's team and in my class. I yelled for the teacher to do something, but all she did was sit down in a corner and cry. She was afraid and did not know what to do.

I tried to get in the middle of the two girls and things only got worse. The girls on Dani's team took the extra balls from the gym office and started throwing them at the girls on the other team. The girls on Casey's team found some footballs and did the same until someone yelled, "STOP!" I guess that must have been me. At first no one listened, but when they realized what had happened, they all stood still and no one moved.

I could not believe it. Lying in the middle of the floor was Genesis. Her eyes were closed and she looked like she was having trouble breathing. No one moved. I ran out of the gym to the nurse's office and got some help. The gym teacher did nothing. The girls in the seventh grade ran out of the gym at the end of the class and never told anyone what had happened, leaving the girls in my class to take the blame and have to explain to the adults how Genesis got hurt.

The nurse came and said that she had a weak pulse and that she was unconscious. She tried to revive her using smelling salts, but it did not work. She called an ambulance from the phone in the gym and we prayed it would come fast.

When it finally arrived and they had taken her to the hospital and contacted her parents, the rest of us knew that the trouble had only just begun. The girls in the seventh grade blamed us for what happened to Genesis.

They said we were playing too rough and that one of us started the fight and tripped Kati Rose and Carly Megan, even though we all knew that it was Genesis. The principal came, took all of us to his office, and told us that some or all of us would be suspended for what happened to her. Kati Rose and Carly Megan both said that Mary Rose and Josie J threw one of the extra balls at Genesis, and that was what knocked her out. They never said that it might have been one of their footballs.

Unfortunately, they had made up their minds to believe the tough girls because they were afraid of them, and Mary Rose and Josie J and three other girls in my class were suspended for throwing the extra balls at the other team and injuring Genesis, who had started the whole thing. No one bothered to think that maybe it was just a game, the kids had overreacted, and the adult who was supposed to teach us sportsmanship had done nothing to stop the fight or control the girls in either class.

As a result dodge ball was eliminated from the gym program. The teacher was fired for not doing anything or calling for help. The girls in the seventh grade never got punished, and I was fuming.

The next time we had gym we learned that Genesis would be out of school for a long time with a severe head injury. We learned that for now, both classes would be separated, and everyone would learn the rules for sports-

manship and the consequences for not following them
The new gym teacher was a man who had just retired from
the marines, and no one was going to start with him. His
name was Mr. Robbie and he was really tough. He was
six feet four inches tall with blonde hair, and was really
pumped. No one would mess with him.

But, I was still upset because the girls in my class got
suspended and Dani, Casey and the other girls got away
with what they had done.

*What would you have done if you were Mary Rose or
Joseia J? Their parents and the principal did not even listen to
their side of the story. They just passed judgment.*

*What would you do the next time you meet the girls in the
seventh grade?*

*How would you get justice for your friends? How do you
think you would get the point across and change what had happened to Mary Rose and Josie J?*

*Good sportsmanship is important no matter what you are
playing. Playing fair is important too. Playing to hurt someone
and not caring is wrong, and that's why people get hurt.*

Love,

Bertha

Bertha, JT, The Frogs
and the Skunk

Some kids are curious, and others are just plain too smart for their own good. My little nephew JT is one of those little four-year-old kids that has to know everything and is into everything that he sees. He loves crawling under floorboards in the cellar and hunting for bugs in the woods. He loves going under parked cars to hunt for dropped coins. But, what he especially loves is frogs, all types of frogs. Big ones, little ones, short fat frogs, anything that even resembles or looks like a frog is on his list of things to collect and find. No matter where we are or what we are doing, you have to keep twelve eyes on him because you never know where he will go or what he will get into too.

This brings me to his latest adventure that sent me, Bertha, on a frog hunt in the woods. It all started one morning in the country during summer vacation when JT could not find his latest pet frog, Sam. He had put the frog in a huge can on the back porch of our bungalow in the country. When he got up to go to camp in the morning, Sam was gone. You see, there had been a rash of frog stealing by the little kids, and you really had to make sure that if you had a great frog it was well protected. Some people even suggested that maybe you needed to take out frog insurance in case of theft.

JT had a friend named Jason. They were inseparable, and did everything together, especially frog hunting and frog stealing. They would not let a leaf go unturned, a rock unmoved, or a tree unclimbed when they were looking to find a frog and take it to their bungalow as a pet.

JT was very upset because he did not know what had happened to Sam. So, JT, Jason and their friend Todd decided to go off on their own one morning to find another frog—or rather three more—so that each one would have their very own pet Sam, and would not have to worry that one of them would steal the other's precious frog.

Without making a sound, they quietly left their houses and snuck off into the woods and began looking around for anything that moved and could be captured inside their shirts, put in their pockets or in a sneaker. JT spotted it first. They had walked deep into the woods when they came to a small pond and saw something large and green. It was a really large frog that was just lying there minding its own business until these three decided to disturb it. Looking around they searched for two more frogs and found smaller ones, making each one of them happy to have their own pet frog.

JT, who had spotted the large one first, needed help to get it back to his bungalow, so the other two were going to have to help him. JT and Big Todd decided to each take a side, and poor Jason got the middle. They would take the big frog to Todd's bungalow for the night, to make sure that it was safe. The only problem was they had gone so far into the woods they were lost, and had no idea where they were or how they would get out.

They each thought that they knew the way until they finally realized that they were lost, and it was getting really dark, and the three brave adventurers were getting scared. But, not so scared or so upset that they would even think of letting the poor frogs go back to their pond where they were so happy until they came along.

When JT's mother Myrtle came home from shopping with her friends, she went to call JT in for dinner and a bath. But, she could not find him. Jason and Todd's mother's could not find them either. So, what do these three do, they come yelling for me, Bertha. "Bertha, where are you?" they screamed in unison. "Why don't you know where JT and his friends are?" yelled Myrtle.

I just looked at them in total amazement. Why didn't they know where their kids were, and why blame me? I was eleven years old and went to camp just like the little ones did, and I couldn't watch them every minute of every day. So, they just stood there with their hands on their hips, totally stumped.

Finally, I told them I would go look in the camp house, or better yet, under it. No luck. Then, I realized that JT's pet Sam was missing, and maybe they went off into the woods when no one was looking to find another frog. Well, as luck would have it they decided that was probably where they were, and since they were not dressed for the woods and it was my idea, I got to go and look for them. I took my cell phone with me in case I got lost, and prayed that I would not get eaten by a wild bear, deer or attacked by a skunk while looking for them.

I walked into the woods hoping to find them because I knew that was the only place they could possibly be. As I walked deeper into the woods it started to get darker and darker. The sky looked like it was about to open up and a raging storm would be upon us in no time. I had no sweater, and was wearing just a pair of shorts and a tank top and was starting to shake from the cold, when I heard three little voices yelling and shouting for help at the top of their lungs. One was shivering from the cold, one was trying to rub two stones together to make a fire, and the other was holding the reason they went into the woods in the first place…a huge and warty looking green frog that they named Elvis. Todd had another frog and so did Jason, which they named Sam 2 and Sam 3.

As I walked toward where they were I realized that I did not even know how far I had gone into the woods or where I was. Better yet, I was totally out of breath from climbing over blocked paths and small hills, and I needed to catch my breath before even trying to get all of us out of the woods safely. Weighing over 165 pounds it was difficult to be a hiker, much less walk in the woods over rocky paths and hills. As I was about to sit on what I thought was a huge boulder, I saw it move. It was the largest tortoise I had ever seen, and I had almost crushed it by trying to use it as a resting place.

Next, I saw this thing moving in the woods. It was getting dark and it was hard to see two feet in front of me, so it was all but impossible to see what this thing was. I walked slowly as not to let it know I was there, when all of a sudden it started to spray me, and boy did it stink. Yes, I got skunked. Not only did I get skunked by one skunk, but he had a half a dozen friends with him. I screamed and yelled for help, and the three boys heard me and followed the awful smell to find me sitting on the ground in total shock and crying. How was I supposed to rescue these three kids after being skunked? To make matters even worse, they just stood there laughing at me while holding their frogs.

I wanted to just leave them there and teach them a good lesson, but I knew I would get in trouble and they would be off the hook. So, we started to walk back to the bungalow colony and could not find our way. Plus, I'd dropped my phone trying to cover my eyes and face when the skunks sprayed me.

Jason and JT thought that they might remember some landmark that would help us find our way back. They said they did this all the time and never got lost or even caught. But, this time they saw the big frog, chased it until they caught him and forgot to drop pebbles along the way to find their way back. I guess they thought they were Hansel and Gretel and would be saved somehow, but not by a wicked witch. As we walked in some direction we saw a light shining at us. I could not believe that Jason and JT's dads had actually noticed that they were missing. They had arrived for the weekend and found the three mothers crying because their three angels were missing. When they finally saw us they did not know whether to laugh or cry from the sight of three muddy kids and three unhappy frogs, and one oversized smelly girl who was muddy and skunked. No one wanted to go near me, and I was not allowed in the bungalow until someone poured tomato juice all over me and attempted to get my clothes off —

that's right, outside, for the entire world to see — before allowing me near the bathroom and a tomato juice bath.

What I did not know at the time was that JT had put his frog on the side of the bathtub in a can and it had jumped into the tub with me. I screamed when something was crawling up my leg. I jumped out of the tub, covered in tomato juice, and yelled for help at the top of my lungs. The problem was that my mom was not there and my sister, Tillie, had some friends over, and they came into the bathroom and were hysterically laughing at the sight of me. Imagine my humiliation until someone finally gave me a towel and a robe. I still smelled from skunk, but I had gotten most of the smell out of my hair, and I was going to use soap and bath bubbles to try and get the rest. JT came running, not because of me, but because of Elvis, his frog. He took the frog and put him in the sink and rinsed him off, then put him back in the can until morning.

The next morning, JT decided that since poor Elvis came from the woods, he had no parents to teach him proper hygiene. He had popped out of the can and might have gotten germs from the floor of the bathroom or the grime in the tub. He was more upset because the frog smelled like tomato juice with a touch of skunk perfume. JT decided to give the frog an Ivory Soap and Ivory

Liquid bubble bath. Imagine walking into the bathroom and seeing a four-year-old child standing on a stool with Ivory soap and Ivory liquid for bubbles, giving the frog a bubble bath…it was a funny sight. The frog was hopping around in the water and slipping out of his hands to try and get away. JT was soaking wet, and so was the floor. The poor frog, if it could talk, would have screamed for help. After all, he was happy just being full of dirt and leaves and grime from the forest, and really did not need to take a bath.

When his mother Myrtle went into the bathroom and realized what he was doing, she just stood there and laughed. She laughed so hard that tears were coming down her eyes and her face turned red. She could not move from where she was standing, and just watched him giving this frog a bath and talking to it as if it was a person. When he finished giving it the bath he took a clean bath towel to dry him off and placed him back in a new and clean can with some leaves to eat and other foods he thought frogs liked. Then, he put the frog on the porch of the bungalow and went back inside, got dressed, and went to camp … but not before putting a "DO NOT TOUCH OR MOVE" sign on the can.

When Myrtle and his father JT came back from shopping they heard a loud thump coming from the can. Unfortunately, frogs should not have Ivory soap or liquid baths, and the frog had died. They did not want JT to know this, but they felt they had to tell him because he needed to know for the next time. But they were too chicken to tell him and told me that, since I let him bring the frog from the forest, I should break the news to him.

Why me? Why did poor Bertha, the scapegoat, always get the jobs no one else would want to do? Why should I tell this four-year-old curious and impish little guy that his frog died because of something he did? This could scar him for life. So, I had a plan. I would go back into the woods with one of my friends and get a new frog for him before he came home from camp. This would mean I would have to invent an excuse to get out of going to camp myself. I told everyone that my grandmother needed me to pick some blueberries for her to use in a pie she was making for company this weekend, and I was the only one she trusted with that job.

I went back into the woods wearing rain gear, carrying an umbrella and wearing a hairnet, rain bonnet and anything else that would protect me from getting skunked again. I asked my cousin, Annie, to come with me because I did not want to take a chance and get lost again. I remembered to take a cell phone with me and a whistle to blow in case we could not find our way back.

We went into the woods and went about half way in before we found another frog. This one looked just like

Elvis, but was a little smaller. I decided I would tell JT that the frog got smaller because he washed him and dried him. I hoped that he would believe me, otherwise the truth was a good idea, I guessed. We picked him up and put him in a pail that I had filled with water, and hoped that he would not hop around too much. I did not want to take a chance and suffocate the poor frog.

We got back to the bungalow unnoticed, and I slipped Elvis the second inside the same can as Elvis the first and hoped JT would not realize it.

When he came home from camp he went for the frog, looked at him and started to play with it on the porch. He brought the frog over to Jason's bungalow and never realized it was not the same one.

Lessons Learned:

- Never give a frog a bath with anything.
- Get your pets from a pet store or from a shelter.
- Make sure that you understand how to take care of your pet no matter what kind of pet it is.
- Make sure you speak to a professional before buying a pet and ask questions about proper care for the pet and food.
- Make sure you know where this pet should sleep.

- Make sure you understand that you are responsible for your own pet.
- Be kind to your pet.
- Give it a good home.

Love,

Bertha

The Contest

I'm never doing my homework again. I am never going back to that class with that miserable old witch of a teacher. She is a poor excuse for something, but I don't know exactly what. I am not going to clean my room ever again, and my sister better not try and come in here. I am on strike, and no one and I mean no one better try and come into this room. I am going to put my bed in front of the door and I am on a total strike! Changes must be made before I will agree to come out ever again. It's a good thing that I have all the candy and junk food I need to keep me from starving and wasting away.

This is a story of what happened when I, Bertha finally could not take it any more.

Throwing my books on the floor of my room and slamming the door shut, I, Bertha then took all of the things on my bed and started throwing them all over the place. Then I unmade my bed, stomped on everything on the floor, and then proceeded to do the same thing on my sister's side of the room. I was fuming. I was tired of being called fat, tubby and klutzy. I was tired of everyone laughing at me for the way I looked, and I had made up my mind to do something about it.

It all started after lunch in class that day when my teacher asked all of the students to read our fire prevention stories. One of these would be sent to the mayor's office to be entered in the Bronx Borough contest on fire prevention, for the best original ideas on fire prevention. Steve read his first, to be followed by Pamela, Frieda, Donna and several other students whose compositions lacked form, proper grammar and original ideas. Next, Iris, Marcia, and Annie read their compositions.

My story, whose ideas were original, interesting and well written, went last. The class voted that it should be sent to represent the class and the school. However, my teacher, Ms. Rosen, had other ideas and decided to express them in front of the entire class. She really didn't care if she embarrassed me, or hurt my feelings. My aunt was a teacher in the same school, and Ms. Rosen told the class that she had given me the ideas to write the story before coming to school.

I looked at her, stared right into her face, and turned beet red. The other students defended me and that said I, Bertha, had written the story in class, and completed it alone. Everyone in the class had gone home and discussed the stories with their families to get ideas, in order to win the contest for the school and the $1,000 dollars they would get for their school's library. A special pizza party for everyone in the school and a trip to the Metropolitan Museum of Art was their incentive to have someone from the school win.

I could not breathe. I started to shake and got really white. But, not this time, not ever again. I turned around to the teacher and said in a loud voice, "You have been picking on me all year, you old bag. You have been yelling at me because I can't walk as fast as the other kids or race in the gym. You even make fun of me because I am overweight and have trouble walking up to the fifth floor everyday without huffing and puffing. But, the one thing you can never accuse me of is cheating or using anyone else's knowledge to complete an assignment. My classmates and you saw me write this story in class without any notes or ideas written on any papers. You are the ugliest, meanest and cruelest excuse for a teacher I have ever seen."

I got sent to the principal's office, and did not care. It was the first time I had ever really gotten in trouble and I knew that he would call my mother, Rosie. As I stomped out of the room, my foot got caught in a chair and I fell, but no one laughed. They could not believe that I had finally had enough.

I walked into the principal's office, slammed down in a chair, and said nothing. His secretary told me to wait until he called my mother, spoke to the teacher and was ready to discuss the problem. I just glared at all of them. I'd had enough of the teacher picking on me, and I'd had enough of everyone laughing at me for the way I looked. I was not going to take it any more. On top of that, my mother even had the nerve to expect me to clean her room on a Friday, when I wanted to spend some time with my friends, not cleaning with my sister Tillie. I would show them just who would win this argument, and it would not be the adults this time — it would be me, Bertha. By the time I would get done explaining what had happened I would make that old battleaxe apologize to me, and in front of the class too.

I sat on the bench in front of the principal's office and was really fuming. I would rat out that mean old witch to him. He would definitely fire her for not entering my composition in the contest and for embarrassing me in front of my class. When he came out he just stared at me in total disbelief. "I spoke to your teacher and she told me you were very fresh and rude to her. She told me that you even called her names and insulted her in front of the class. Is that true, Bertha?" I just glared at him and said nothing. I knew that if I spoke I would only make it worse. So, I just sat there and said not a word.

The principal, Mr. Greenhouse, just stood there with his hands folded in front of him, waiting for me to answer when his secretary came out and said my mother had arrived. Oh, great! Now everyone in the whole world will know that I, Bertha, was in trouble because my mother was here in school, and she just had to drag my sister, Tillie, with her. Tillie was sitting on the bench and gloating because I was in trouble for talking back to the teacher, and she knew that I would be grounded forever.

My mother did not say anything to me while the principal was telling her the teacher's side of the story. I was fuming because he left out how rude she was to me and the real reason why I was disrespectful to her and why I got angry. Ms. Rosen did not like my aunt, who also taught sixth grade, and was jealous of her because her students really liked her and none of Ms. Rosen's did. She was also angry because the principal always asked my aunt to supervise the musical productions and not her. My sister, Tillie, was going to be the star in the production of *Carousel* and I might be allowed to play the piano for some of the selections. No one bothered to tell my mom about the contest regarding fire prevention, and why I'd stormed out of the room in anger.

I sat there as long as I could listening to them talk about me as if I wasn't there. My mom, who formed an opinion and never changed it, decided that I must be wrong and never gave me a chance to speak. That is wrong…kids should be able to defend themselves, and they have rights too! But, no one ever listened to me. I was supposed to be Bertha the Perfect and never question anyone and just go along with whatever the adults said or did. I was not going to sit there and take it this time!

I got up, stood on top of the bench, and told everyone to be quiet in my loudest voice. They all just looked at me in total surprise. I was not going to go down for something that was not my fault. I probably could have told the teacher how I felt about her in a better way, but being a kid — and kids have outbursts and can't always express themselves the way adults think they should — I did it my way.

"Mom, Principal Greenspan — and even you Tillie — just be quiet and listen to me for a change," said Bertha. "I did nothing wrong. That teacher decided my outstanding composition on fire prevention would not be entered in the mayor's contest on fire safety because she said that my aunt helped me write it. That is as much as saying that I cheated on a test and got a perfect score because I copied someone's answers." I felt that my character and ethics were being attacked and that I was being wrongly accused of something that I would never do. I also felt that she was mean to me, and had always made me feel unwanted in her class by commenting on my weight, how I looked, and the way I walked. I felt that she was mean, awful and should not be allowed to get away with that kind of behavior towards her students.

They all just stood there, shook their heads and said nothing. I walked out of his office, left the building, and went straight home to face my punishment and the wrath of my mother and father for whatever it was I was supposed to have done.

When I got home I decided to make a real statement and went about destroying my room. I would never clean it again, nor would I ever do homework or enter a stupid contest.

I locked the door and refused to allow anyone in. My sister wanted to talk to me, but I told her to get lost. My grandmother, who was the only one that I trusted, told them all to leave me alone and let me calm down on my own.

I decided that I was going to write up a list of rules and a contract for everyone in my family to follow. I would even make one up for my class and give it to the principal before I would agree to go back to school ever again. Just like teachers have codes of conduct for their students to follow with rewards and consequences, I, Bertha, thought that adults and teachers needed some too.

I sat and thought about what to write and how I would finally make my point. If this didn't work I would take drastic measures and take my case to the news, or even send my story to the mayor.

I finally had two sets of rules and posted them on the walls of my room and finally in the kitchen of our apartment. I called everyone together for a family meeting and told them what I thought they needed to do in order for everyone to be treated equally and fairly.

Bertha's Code of Family Conduct:

- Never yell at anyone; it solves nothing, it just gives you a sore throat.

- Listen to someone before accusing them of doing something wrong. There are two sides and you need to listen to both before passing sentence.

- Never — EVER — make fun of someone because of the way they look or if they are different.

- Never laugh when someone cannot do something as well as you can.

- Never ever make fun of someone's clothes or shoes or hairdo.

- Be respectful to adults and be respectful to children too. To get respect you need to give it.

- Never accuse someone of cheating just because someone said they did.

- Trust your children to tell the truth and they always will.

- Give your child a hug before going to bed and going to school.

- Do not punish your child just because someone says they did something wrong. If your child is usually good, have faith that maybe the other person is not telling the truth.

- Talk out all problems before they get worse.

- Remember to say I LOVE YOU to your child no matter what and they will say it to you.

My parents read the rules and they realized that maybe they should have listened to me before grounding me for a month for what happened in school.

I then showed them the rules for listening to students in school and my mother and father agreed to help me by bringing me to school the next day and showing the principal what I had written.

Bertha's Rules of Respect For Students and Teachers:

- Never yell at a student in front of others. Never punish a student without getting all of the facts and listening to both sides.

- Do not embarrass anyone because of how they look, walk or because they are overweight.

- Never accuse someone of cheating unless you can really prove it. It is wrong to prejudge someone because you do not like someone they are related to.

- Talk with the child in private to discuss the problem.

- Be respectful to your students and they will give you respect too.

- Do not let other students make fun of anyone. It is hurtful and rude.

- Let the child or children know that you care about them.

- Children will not all be perfect and sometimes they need extra help; that is why you are there.

- Do not be so quick to pass judgment and give out consequences.

- Making children feel that they are not smart or as smart as other children is not right. Every child should want to come to school and should feel he or she can learn.

I cannot tell you whether Ms. Rosen changed as a result of these rules. I can tell you that my family heard what I said and agreed with my family rules. As for the principal, he was impressed with the fact that I stood up for myself. He did not fire Ms. Rosen, but he did put me in another sixth grade class.

Remember: Children are special people, and they have feelings too. We are all human, and sometimes say things without thinking. But, educators have a special privilege and a special job; they get to teach our most precious diamonds—our children. Children need to know you care. They need structure, discipline and love.

Respect is a two way street. Remember that.

Love, Bertha

Life As I See It

By Fran Lewis

This story is dedicated to my mom, Ruth Swerdloff, who has Alzheimer's and who I love dearly. We pray for a cure for her each day. I think that everyone needs to understand how it feels to live with someone with this disease as both an adult and a child.

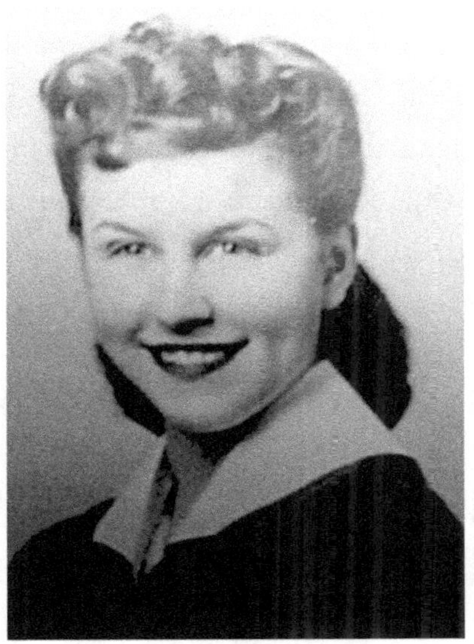

Fran's mother.

Bertha's Grandmother —
Life Through Her Eyes As She Sees It

My name is Bertha and I am now twelve years old. I live with my parents, my sister, Tillie, and my grandparents. My grandma Katie has always been an inspiration to me. Whenever I needed someone to talk to she was the one person who would set me straight, protect me from getting punished, and always understand how difficult it was, and still is, for me to lose weight. I am still quite overweight and I still hate dancing school and ice-skating, but what I hate more is what happened to my grandmother.

It all began one morning when she went out to go to the bakery to buy bread for lunch for my grandfather. My grandfather and I always liked to eat lunch together. I would sit on his lap and share an entire freshly baked rye bread with him — it was the highlight of my day. My grandfather was a very bright and amazing man. He owned a cleaning store on Mohegan Avenue in the Bronx, and I loved going there after school to watch him sew. He was a European tailor and could make anything and anyone look great when he was finished.

On this particular day my grandmother set out to go to the bakery and did not return for quite some time. As she was walking down Tremont Avenue toward the bakery she made a wrong turn. Instead of going straight for three blocks, she turned down the wrong block and wound up on Elsmere Place, and never got to the bakery. Fortunately, an old friend saw her and brought her home. She could not remember where she was going or how she had wound up on Elsmere Place. When she got home she said that she was distracted by something while she was walking and did not realize that she went the wrong way. She made light of it and would not let anyone make a fuss or think anything was wrong.

The next day she started out for the butcher to shop for meat for the Sabbath and the same thing happened, except this time she wound up in front of my grandfather's store and told him she was there for him to take her out to lunch. That is when we realized that something was really wrong. My grandfather came home for lunch every day and he would never eat in a restaurant unless the food was kosher. There were several places in the area that were, but he enjoyed going home for lunch. When she went into the store and told him why she was there, he pretended to agree with her not to embarrass her or create a scene. When he got her home she told him she was sure that she was supposed to meet him for lunch and he was making a big deal out of nothing. That same day she forgot where she put her glasses, her meat grinder and several other things that were right in front of her at the time.

When I came home from school that day and asked her why she was sitting in the kitchen just staring at the stove, she told me she was thinking about what to make for dinner that night. She started to go over to the stove and prepare the meat and potatoes that she had taken out, and placed them on a low flame to cook. I went into my room to do my homework and forgot about what she was doing until I smelled something burning. I ran out of my room followed by my sister, Tillie, and what we saw was so frightening we could not believe it. The food in the pot was burnt, the flame had been turned up too high, and food was splattering all over the floor and the ceiling. My grandmother just stood there and stared, and had no idea what was happening or why.

I called my mom, Rosie, who called our family doctor to come for a house call. When he arrived he quietly took my grandmother into her room and did an exam plus some other things with memory and coordination. Our family doctor was amazing. He could diagnose anything and was never wrong. He told us that she needed some more tests to be taken in a diagnostic lab, but that he was fairly certain that she had what was called dementia. This was a memory problem where the person started to forget things, like where they put certain objects, the days of the week, how to write or read, or even where they lived. It was a slow moving disease that turned into Alzheimer's, and there was no cure. They could give her certain medications, but the disease had a mind of its own and no one could stop it.

After taking the tests at the lab we found out that she'd had a mini stroke and that was part of the problem. Unfortunately, she was only going to get worse. I, Bertha, was determined to make sure that I learned as much about this disease as possible so that I could help her in order to make sure that she stayed at home and not anywhere else.

I learned that she might get violent or even use bad language as her behavior changed. I learned that she might not remember that she ate, and might even say and do things that would be out of character. I learned that we had to watch her and make sure that she did not leave the house alone or wander out by herself.

Each day I would go to school, but not before checking on her and making sure that she would be safe all day. My parents, my grandfather, and my aunt took turns staying home and taking care of her. This was a hard job. Grandma Katie was someone who took care of everyone and was the glue that held everyone together, so it was hard for me and everyone else to see her this way.

Things got even worse. She started to have accidents and needed to wear Pampers like little children do. She did not remember that she had to go to the bathroom, and did not know that she had gone at all. She started to sit in her reclining chair and watch television all day, but could not tell you what she watched or who was in the program.

When I came home from school and finished my homework, I would sit and watch with her and explain what the show was about, or read her a story so that she might understand something that was going on around her. I guess I could only hope and pray. When our doctor came the next time, he suggested that my family think about getting some help at home to make life easier for everyone. My grandfather got someone to come for a few hours a day to take care of her while everyone was at work. But I was worried about a stranger taking care of her and started to pretend to be sick so I could stay home from school and take care of her myself. My sister, Tillie, did the same thing, and at least two days a week one of us faked illness to help out. I think my parents knew what we were doing, but never stopped us from staying home. Even though the people that came to take care of her were nice and kind, they were not us. You need family around to make sure that the person is okay and treated the right way.

It has been many years now since Grandma got sick. She got worse, but she is still at home and has twenty-four hour care. My grandfather is gone. So, it is up to the rest of us to take care of her. She knows who we are and she understands when it is time to eat, or if she is too hot or too cold. She knows her name, but she does not know the day of the week or the month of the year. But, she is here, and maybe someday there will be a cure.

If my grandmother could tell you her story this is what she would say:

My day starts when I open my eyes and find myself sleeping on my chair. I try to get up but someone stops me. I jump at the sound of the person's voice, and become very scared and frightened. I usually start to scream, "Get out of my house, why are you here?" Then, I use some profanities and start telling people to leave my house and leave me alone. Finally, I cry so hard and so uncontrollably that I begin to shake. All the while this person is trying to calm me down and tells me, "Katie, everything will be okay. It's me, Joan; you know me. I love you."

Joan stands in front of me and I really don't know her name or anyone else's for that matter, but I do know her face. Then, my day begins with her taking me to the bathroom and helping me get cleaned up. I smell something and realize that I soiled my diaper, and I am not capable of changing it. I try to tell her that but it comes out like, "I know you did it, I think so too, just do it. Don't you remember?" That seems to be what I say a lot of the time. I don't know why.

After getting cleaned up she takes me into another place and gives me food. I have no idea what she is giving me or what you call it. I look at it and she says it is called oatmeal. It could be anything and I would not know it. She could give me dog food or worse and I would still eat it if I felt hungry. The trouble is … I can't remember what I was going to say. I started to tell her the oatmeal was no good but I cannot tell her why. I just stare out into space and forget that I was even eating anything at all. She asks me what is no good and I begin shouting, "NO GOOD! NO GOOD! NO GOOD!" and throw the spoon at her, and it lands on the floor. I think she is about to say something when my daughter walks in and sees what happened. She looks at me covered in oatmeal and the food all over the floor, and asks Joan what caused me go get so agitated. I am trying to say that the oatmeal was too hot, but I cannot remember what hot means, or that it needed some sugar because I like things sweeter.

My daughter looks at me and just smiles. I know everything will be okay because she is there. She came to give me something that looked like a lot of things, but I don't know why I have to take them or if I will even like them. Some look like candy, some look like round things, and the rest look like mush. She calls it my medicine and says that I need to take these things in order to be okay. I just spit them all out and yell, "NO!"

Then all of a sudden something strange that has never happened before really puts me over the edge. I start to curse and use all kinds of bad words and cannot stop myself. I keep telling whoever the fat lady is that is in my house to, "Get out you fat thing and never come back!"

She stays calm, and just says, "Katie, we all love you, it will be okay."

I just glare at her in total horror and start to try and leave. "I am not staying here with you. You can't make me. I hate you." I am ranting like a crazy lady and cannot stop. All of a sudden someone else comes and both of them just look at me and don't know whether to laugh or cry. I just … I don't know what I did. I went back to sleep on my chair and let them worry about what to do.

When I wake up again I do not remember what happened before, but I know something in me has changed. I begin talking funny and sound like something out of a horror movie, yelling, "WOO WOO WOO WOO," and waving my arms as if I am possessed. As I start smiling strangely, I hear the two of them say I sound like I think I am a different person, trying out different voices, but I have no idea what they are talking about. I start to pretend I am dancing and say, "I want to float and fly over there with the birds. Don't you see them?" Then I say, "I want to go over there and eat and eat all of you." I cannot control my words or what I am saying.

I become so out of control that Joan has to call my neighbor and my daughter to stop me from yelling and screaming. All I keep saying is, "Don't you remember, leave me alone, get out of here and stop trying to kill me!" I start to speak, but no one knows it's me. I sound like three different people, and they think I am going crazy.

Throughout the day the same things happen until I get an extra dose of medication to help control my outbursts and calm me down. Even the doctor does not know what to say when they call him. His words are, "That is the disease progressing; get used to it." Get used to what, not knowing who I am or who anyone else is? I do not even know my own daughter who is standing next to me and trying her best to stay calm for my benefit.

What happens next is earthshaking and worse. All of a sudden the aide sees something brown and awful on the carpet when she helps me to the table to eat something. It runs down my legs, and I cannot control it or stop it from coming. It looks like a river of dark chocolate. She just shakes her head and takes me to the bathroom, and does her best not to get upset. The rug, her shoes, and the carpet are one big mess and smell, not to mention me. I start to cry because I know that I did something bad. I say, "I am bad; I am sorry. Don't yell at me." Of course no one does.

When it gets dark I get scared because I can't tell the difference between day and night. I just sit in my chair and watch whatever is on that thing in front of me. Sometimes I talk to the people on that thing and start yelling at them. If I see someone on it hurting someone, I think it is really happening. If I see something I don't like I start screaming and yelling for someone to change it.

Life has not been the same for me for over four years. It will probably only get worse. My children say I am going to be eighty years old on Thanksgiving Day. I don't even know what that means. All I say when they tell me I am going to my son's for that day is, "Okay." Then, "I want my son, I want him now. No one else cares about me, just him." I guess I say that because he is always working and I really never see him except when I imagine it in my dreams. I see a lot of people in my dreams. I see my husband and my sister, who are not here anymore. I see my brothers too. I talk to myself, and sometimes I even talk to pictures on the piano and to that thing in front of me.

When am I going to be myself again? When is someone going to be able to help me? I think the answer is NEVER!

How would you like to live each day like this?

— Katie

I wrote this story from Bertha to everyone to make you understand how important it is to care for someone with this disease. It is an awful disease and anyone can get it. I love my mom and she is home with twenty-four hour care. Thanks to the people at Partner's In Care who provide the aides. Thanks to the four best home health aides who are part of our family: Joan, Pat, Joyce and Gail. We love you, and so does Ruth.

Love,

Fran and Bertha